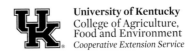

University of Kentucky
College of Agriculture,
Food and Environment
Cooperative Extension Service

Cook Together, Eat Together

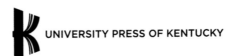

UNIVERSITY PRESS OF KENTUCKY

Cooperative Extension Service | Agriculture and Natural Resources | Family and Consumer Sciences | 4-H Youth Development | Community and Economic Development

Editorial and Sales Offices: The University Press of Kentucky
663 South Limestone Street, Lexington, Kentucky 40508-4008
www.kentuckypress.com

Acknowledgments

This material was funded by USDA's SNAP. USDA is an equal opportunity provider and employer.

Authors:

Rebecca Freeman, Social Marketing Project Manager

Jackie Walters, MBA, RDN, Extension Specialist

Janet Mullins, PhD, RDN, Extension Specialist

Jean Najor, MS, Cooperative Extension Service Nutrition Education Program

Anita Courtney, MS, Consultant for Social Marketing

Design and Layout:

Kevin Brumfield, Graphic Designer

Photographs:

Pablo Alcala, Photojournalist

Copy Editing and Proofreading:

Vickie Mitchell, Editor

Educational programs of Kentucky Cooperative Extension serve all people regardless of race, color, age, sex, religion, disability or national origin.

CONTENTS

CONTENTS

Cook Together, Eat Together

Never Underestimate the Power of a Good Meal

If you want to bring your family together, the kitchen is a good place to start. Cooking and eating together is a great way to build family closeness. But when budgets are tight, it is a challenge to put a meal on the table. We hope this book makes that process easier and more enjoyable.

To create this book, we listened to people who are experts on this topic, mothers across Kentucky who are SNAP (Supplemental Nutrition Assistance Program) eligible and who know how to stretch a dollar to feed their families.

Though it is a challenge to cook when funds are limited, having good basic cooking skills makes it easier. Kentucky moms told us about friends who "can throw down in the kitchen" and "who can make something from nothing." They said their kids became more independent and confident when they helped out in the kitchen. Families also found it was fun to cook together, as a team, and that cooking teaches many skills—from organization to math.

Kentucky mothers said that learning to cook well boosted their confidence and reduced their stress. And, when the cooking was done, families found they looked forward to sitting down to a home-cooked meal together.

The topics we have covered and the types of recipes we chose were based on things that real people told us would be helpful. Comments from the mothers we talked with are in quotation marks throughout the book so you can share in their humor and learn from their wisdom.

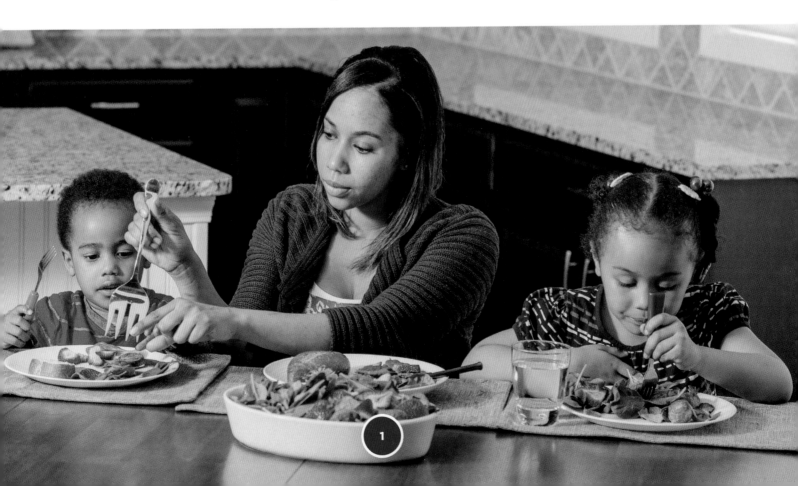

Basics for Healthy Eating on a Budget

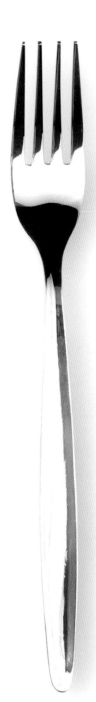

Best Buys. Dried beans, eggs, cabbage, bananas, cornmeal and oatmeal are among the most nutritious foods for the money. Learn to make delicious foods with these basics.

Eat Smaller Portions. Eat less, spend less, weigh less. Serve smaller portions at dinner and you may have enough for lunch the next day. Big muffins can be split in half. One half cup is a serving size for rice, noodles and cereals; but many people eat a cup or two. A serving of meat is 3 ounces, about the size of a deck of cards. One way to eat less is to serve food on smaller plates—it makes the portions appear bigger.

Waste Not. Americans throw away roughly 30 million tons of food each year. Before you put perishables in your grocery cart, think about how and when you'll use them. When you buy perishables, wrap them well so they stay fresher longer. When vegetables become slightly wilted and are not good for a salad, use them in a soup, stew or omelet.

Think Frozen. With frozen foods, you can use the amount you need, reseal the bag and reduce waste. Use plain frozen vegetables. Vegetables frozen in butter sauce cost twice as much and have far more calories.

Go Generic. Buy store brands instead of pricier national brands. Many grocery companies buy national-brand products and put their own label on them.

Less Meat. Try serving smaller portions of meat; extend the meal by serving more whole grains, beans and vegetables.

Buy Produce in Season. Check the grocery ads in your newspaper to find the week's best buys. Many Kentucky farmers markets accept SNAP benefits.

Use Sales and Coupons. Planning meals around what's on sale can lower your grocery bills, especially if you also use coupons. Just make sure they're for items you would buy anyway.

Brown-Bag It. Packing lunch is a great way to save money and an excellent use of leftovers.

Plan Ahead. Shopping with specific meals in mind for the week ahead makes it easier to buy in bulk and repurpose ingredients. For example, turn Sunday night's roast chicken into Monday night's enchiladas. The more you cook from scratch, the further your dollar can stretch.

Water First. Don't buy sodas and other drinks. Make water your main beverage, and watch your food costs and calories drop. American families spend on average $850 a year on soft drinks. Tap water costs a penny a gallon. Drink water first.

Buying Spices Can Be Pricey. Spices seem expensive but because you use small amounts of them, they go a long way. Consider buying one spice a month. If you can shop at ethnic markets, you may be able to find good deals on spices.

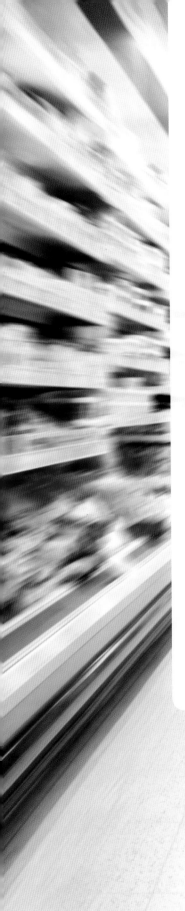
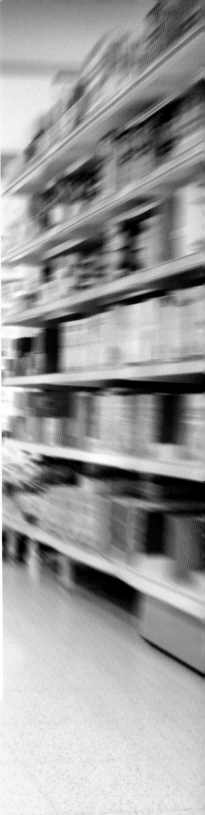

Shop Smart
at Grocery Stores

Buying healthy food on a tight budget can be a challenge, but the more you know, the easier it is to buy nutritious foods without exceeding your budget. Here are some tips to help you get healthier food at a better price.

Before you go

To stay within your budget, plan meals and make a shopping list before you go to the store. For example, if you plan to make spaghetti for dinner on Tuesday and tacos on Thursday, your menu might keep you from making a pricey impulse purchase that is not a part of your plan.

Store layout

Learn the facts about store layout. Grocery stores are designed to encourage shoppers to spend the most money. A few facts:

◆ **Look low for lower prices.** Stores put generic and less-expensive items below eye-level, typically on the bottom shelf, because they make less money on them.

◆ **Don't assume that products in end-of-aisle displays are bargains.** They are often put there to get your attention and to move products fast.

◆ **Look for Manager's Specials.** They are usually good deals and are often marked with bright stickers or signs.

◆ **Be savvy about the tricks of the trade.** Child-oriented products — snacks and cereals — are placed at children's eye level. Grocers know that children often talk their parents into buying things. Skip those aisles or be ready to set limits if you're shopping with your children.

Unit Pricing: The key to smart shopping

Compare the cost of products by using unit pricing. Have you ever looked at a box of cereal that is on sale and wondered if it was really a good deal? One of the most helpful tools in the grocery store is unit prices. These are the small codes on the shelf below the product that show how much something costs per unit (ounce, pound). Unit pricing allows you to easily compare brands and package sizes to find the best deal for your money. The unit prices below show that Snappy Rice Cereal is seven cents cheaper per ounce than Crackly Rice Cereal. Unit pricing is not available in all stores or on all items.

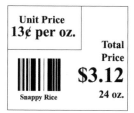
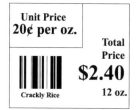

Food Labels

Using the sample label at right, check out ① **Servings Per Container** and ② **Serving Size** to see how large a serving is and how many people the product will serve. For example, if there are 2 servings listed and you eat the whole container, you're eating double the calories on the label.

The ③ **% Daily Value** column lists percentages based on recommended daily allowances based on a 2,000 calorie per day diet. For example, a label may show that a serving of the food provides 30 percent of the daily recommended amount of fiber. This means you may need another 70 percent to meet the recommended goal. Remember, this is just an estimate, but it serves as a good guide.

Try to minimize ④ **Saturated Fat** and ⑤ **Trans Fat**. These are both bad fats that clog arteries.

The less ⑥ **Cholesterol** and ⑦ **Sodium** you eat, the better. The latest recommendation for sodium is less than 2,300 mg per day for adults and even less for kids, depending on their age.

In addition, try to keep the amount of ⑧ **added sugars** low since these are sugars and syrups that are added to foods when they are prepared. More sugars means more calories.

Get enough ⑨ **Fiber,** ⑩ **Vitamin D,** ⑪ **Calcium,** ⑫ **Iron,** and ⑬ **Potassium**.

Keep your kids occupied at the store by asking them to read labels. Studying labels will help your family make the best choices.

Nutrition Facts

① 8 servings per container

② **Serving size**   **2/3 cup (55g)**

Amount per serving

Calories   230

% Daily Value* ③

Total Fat 8g	**10%**
Saturated Fat 1g ④	**5%**
Trans Fat 0g ⑤	
Cholesterol 0mg ⑥	**0%**
Sodium 160mg ⑦	**7%**
Total Carbohydrate 37g	**13%**
Dietary Fiber 4g ⑨	**14%**
Total Sugars 12g	
Includes 10g Added Sugars ⑧	**20%**
Protein 3g	

Vitamin D 2mcg ⑩	10%
Calcium 260mg ⑪	20%
Iron 8mg ⑫	45%
Potassium 235mg ⑬	6%

* The % Daily Value (DV) tells you how much a nutrient in a serving of food contributes to a daily diet. 2,000 calories a day is used for general nutrition advice.

⑭   **INGREDIENTS:** MILLED CORN, SUGAR, CORN SYRUP, MOLASSES, SALT, PARTIALLY HYDROGENATED VEGETABLE OIL (ONE OR MORE OF: COCONUT, COTTONSEED, AND SOYBEAN)***†, SODIUM, ASCORBATE AND ASCORBIC ACID (VITAMIN C), NIACINAMIDE, REDUCED IRON, ZINC OXIDE, WHEAT STARCH, PYRIDOXINE HYDROCHLORIDE (VITAMIN B₆), RIBOFLAVIN (VITAMIN B₂), THYAMIN HYDROCHLORIDE (VITAMIN B₁), ANNATTO COLOR, VITAMIN A PALMITATE, BHT (PRESERVATIVE), FOLIC ACID, VITAMIN B₁₂ AND VITAMIN D.
***ADDS A NEGLIGABLE AMOUNT OF FAT.

Scan the **14 ingredients**. Companies are required to list product ingredients on the product's label. Ingredients are listed from the largest amount to the least amount. For example, if sugar is listed first, there is more sugar in the product than any other ingredient. The label at left shows that milled corn is the main ingredient. The next three ingredients are sweeteners: sugar, corn syrup and molasses. When those sweeteners are combined, it may mean there is more sugar than corn in this product.

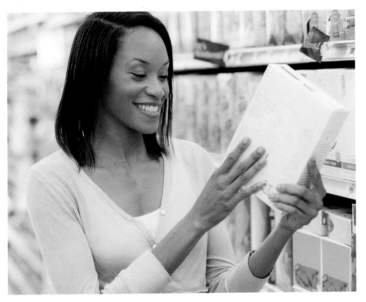

Produce Section

Buy fresh produce in season. Most produce is priced lower when it's in season. Oranges and grapefruit are cheaper and tastier in December and January, the peak of their season. In-season produce is usually displayed at the front of the produce section. Plan your shopping and meals according to what's in season.

Buy the bags. A bag of apples or potatoes is usually cheaper per unit than individual apples or potatoes.

Buy the bargains. Cabbage, potatoes, carrots, bananas and apples are among the most affordable produce.

Buy whole produce. Prepackaged/precut fruits and vegetables usually cost more than whole produce. There are times when prepackaged/precut produce is priced to sell because it tends to have a shorter shelf life, and store managers want to move it quickly.

Use portion power. Serve produce in ½ cup portions to make it go further. A large banana can be split between two kids.

Only buy what you can use. Don't waste produce. Be realistic about how much produce you can prepare and eat before it spoils.

Consider frozen or canned vegetables. If a particular fresh fruit or vegetable is too expensive for your budget, consider buying it frozen or canned.

Bread and Grains

Choose *whole* wheat or *whole* grain bread. Even though a label says "wheat" or "multigrain," the bread isn't always whole wheat or whole grain. Look for "whole wheat" or "whole grain" on the label and in the ingredient list. Whole wheat and whole grain are much more nutritious than white bread.

Don't let any bread go to waste. Stale bread is great for making bread crumbs, croutons and French toast.

Pick cereals with fiber and sugar in mind. Look for cereals with 10 or fewer grams of sugar and 3 or more grams of fiber per serving.

The Meat Department

Just stew it. Stew meat tends to be cheaper per pound than other meats and can be tender and flavorful with long, slow cooking.

Cut it up at home. Boneless, skinless chicken breasts cost much more than a whole chicken. Roasting a whole chicken is easy and when you do cook the whole bird, it can become three meals: roasted chicken, chicken tacos and soup.

When there is **a great sale on meat**, buy extra and freeze it.

Look for **cheaper seafood options** like frozen fish filets.

Dairy Section

Stick with skim or 1% milk. It's cheaper than whole milk and has fewer calories.

Stay away from flavored milks. They're more expensive and have lots of extra sugar that kids develop a taste for. Get them used to drinking white milk.

Consider nonfat dry milk for baking and cooking. Powdered milk is a great bargain. No one will know the difference if you bake or cook with it.

Buy whole cheese instead of shredded or sliced cheese. It usually costs much less per pound.

Buy eggs. They're inexpensive, high in protein and can be made quickly into many satisfying meals.

A few final shopping tips:

Build your pantry by buying one pricey item like olive oil or a spice every other shopping trip. Over time you will have a supply of staples that will enhance the flavor of whatever you prepare.

Don't buy drinks other than milk. Most packaged drinks are overpriced sugar water. Make iced tea (regular or herbal) at home. Add flavor to tea or water with sliced lemons or oranges.

Only use coupons for foods you really need.

Shop Smart at Farmers Markets

Shopping at farmers markets is a great way to get local, delicious produce. Take your kids along. If they haven't already, they may fall in love with fresh fruits and vegetables at the market. Shopping at a farmers' market is a little different than shopping at a grocery store. These tips can help you make the best choices.

◆ **Find a market near you.** Contact your Cooperative Extension office for up-to-date information on farmers markets in your area.

◆ **Find out which markets accept EBT.** Some farmers markets are equipped to accept Electronic Benefit Transfer (EBT) cards from SNAP customers. Some farmers markets offer "double dollars" when people spend their SNAP benefits at the market.

◆ **Know what's in season.** Your mouth might be watering for fresh tomatoes but in most cases, Kentucky-grown tomatoes don't appear at farmers markets until late June. (See the Appendix for the Kentucky Proud Produce Availability Calendar.)

◆ **Look before you buy.** Rather than being swept away by the first ear of corn you see, walk the entire market to see what's available before you make any purchases. You might find that one vendor's prices are lower than the others or that there is better-looking corn a few stands away.

◆ **Ask questions.** Farmers are usually happy to answer questions about their fruits and vegetables. They often have great cooking and serving suggestions.

◆ **Bring the kids.** Let each of them pick out one item. Next thing you know, they may be asking to grow a garden.

◆ **Don't expect a perfect appearance.** Some produce at farmers markets has personality. These vegetables and fruits are usually grown for taste, not appearance. You may find that the produce doesn't look perfect — a slightly off-center pepper or an apple with a rough skin — but it tastes fantastic.

◆ **Ask for seconds.** Sometimes a farmer will have a basket of perfectly good produce that doesn't look good enough to put out at the stand. Ask farmers if they have seconds that they are willing to sell at a reduced rate. You may have to cut a few spots out of a potato but it could be well worth it.

◆ **Go late.** For the best deals, go to the farmers' market late. Farmers often prefer to sell products at a discount rather than load them up and take them home. Keep in mind selling home-grown products is a farmer's livelihood, so don't expect deep discounts.

◆ **Keep it simple.** Since the produce you are buying is super fresh, let its natural flavor show when you prepare it. Keep preparation simple. You'll make cooking easier, and you'll be likely to try (and eat) even more local foods from the farmers' market next week. Sliced tomatoes with a little salt, a fresh apple with peanut butter or roasted potatoes are as good as it gets.

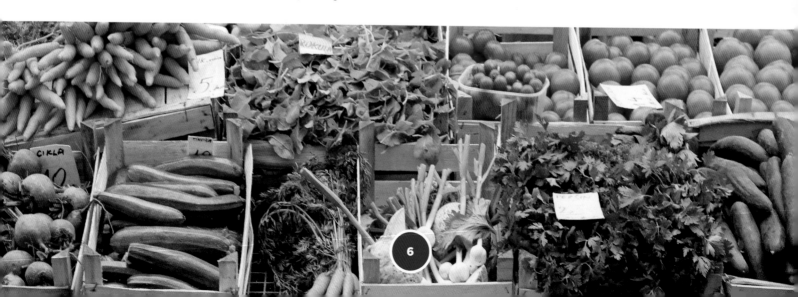

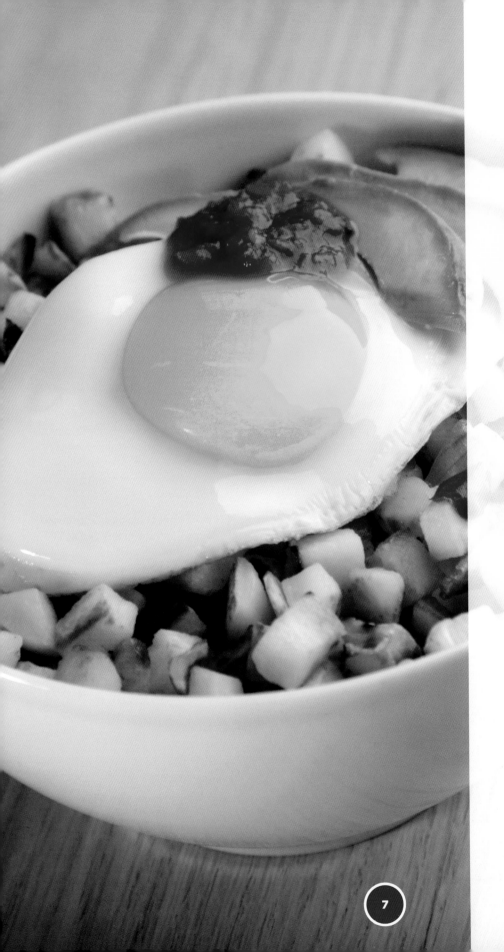

Breakfast

Did you know that people who eat a healthy breakfast of lean protein and/or whole grains are more likely to be at a healthy weight than those who skip it? A healthy breakfast revs up your metabolism and keeps you from overeating later in the day. Kids also benefit from eating breakfast. Children who eat breakfast perform better in the classroom and on the playground. When you eat breakfast, you become a good role model for your kids.

On days when there's no time for a family dinner, consider getting up a few minutes earlier to have a quick breakfast together. Even if your family eats together in the car as you head out to start your day, you are still sharing family time. This time together can help kids feel more secure as they embark on their day.

The tasty, affordable breakfasts we've developed have three themes. All Things Oats offers two recipes, with several variations, that use a grain that is cheap, hearty and tasty. Easy Eggs provides three delicious recipes for one of the most affordable, nutritious and versatile foods. Finally, Grab and Go breakfast ideas allow you and your children to reach for something easy to eat on the way out the door.

INGREDIENTS:

- ½ cup water
- Pinch of salt
- 1½ cups old-fashioned oats
- 1 teaspoon ground cinnamon
- ¼ teaspoon ground nutmeg
- 2 tablespoons brown sugar
- ½ teaspoon vanilla extract
- 1½ cups low-fat milk

Cinnamon Roll Oatmeal

MAKES 4 SERVINGS • SERVING SIZE: ¾ CUP

Hot oatmeal is a great morning comfort food. This recipe uses cinnamon, brown sugar and vanilla to create the flavor of a cinnamon roll. Try the variations we suggest here or create your own.

VARIATIONS:

Berry Cheesecake Oatmeal: Mix in fresh or frozen berries and 1 tablespoon low-fat cream cheese after oatmeal has cooked.

Monkey Meal: Add sliced banana and 1 tablespoon peanut butter when stirring in other ingredients.

Apple Pie Oatmeal: Mix in raisins, walnuts, maple syrup and chopped apples when stirring in other ingredients.

DIRECTIONS:

Stovetop: In a medium saucepan, bring water and salt to a boil. Stir in oats, cinnamon, nutmeg, brown sugar, vanilla extract and milk. Reduce heat and simmer, uncovered, for 5 minutes, stirring occasionally.

Microwave: In a microwave-safe bowl, stir together oats, cinnamon, nutmeg, brown sugar and salt. Stir in water, vanilla extract and milk until well combined. Microwave about 3-5 minutes or until oats are desired consistency.

 Kid Friendly: Help kids arrange fixings the night before for easy assembly in the morning. This teaches them how to plan and makes everyone's life easier.

 Less Mess: To prevent sticking, spray bowl or saucepan with nonstick cooking spray before you add oatmeal.

 Family Time Around the Table: Even if you can't eat together every morning, be sure to acknowledge every family member with a smile, a kind word and a hug.

 Love Those Leftovers: Store leftover oatmeal in the refrigerator. For no-cook refrigerated oatmeal, put ingredients in a jar, put a lid on the jar and shake to combine. Place the jar in the fridge overnight. The oatmeal will keep for up to two days.

 Nice Price: Buy oatmeal in bulk rather than individual packages.

"When you do your own cooking you can satisfy your own taste buds."

NUTRITION FACTS PER SERVING: 180 calories, 2.5g total fat, 0g saturated fat, 0mg cholesterol, 50mg sodium, 32g carbohydrate, 3g dietary fiber, 11g sugar, 9g protein

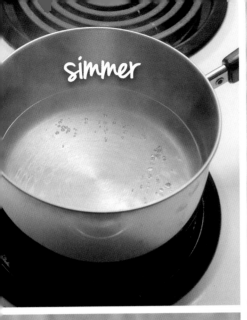
simmer

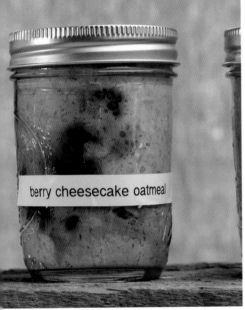
berry cheesecake oatmeal

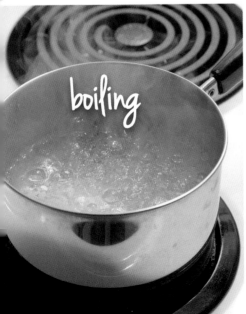
boiling

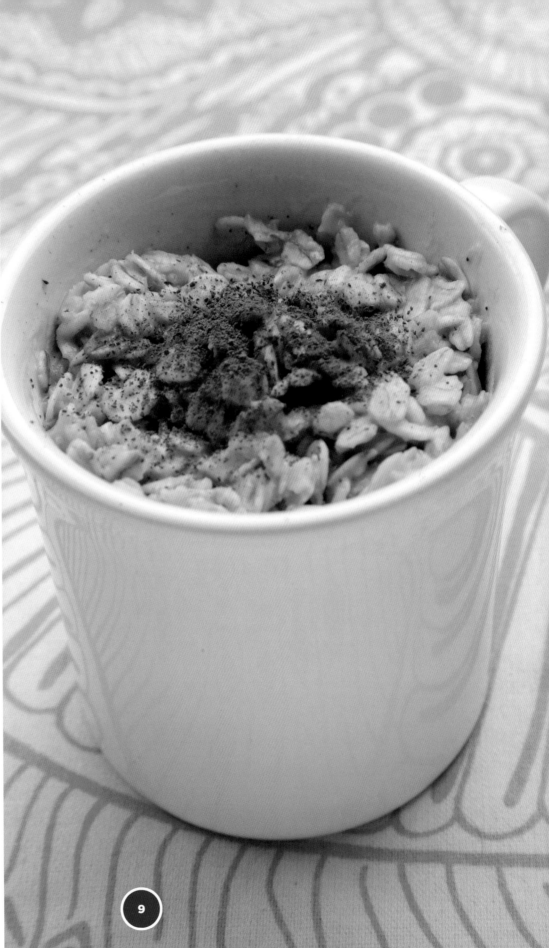

INGREDIENTS:

    Nonstick spray or oil

2   tablespoons + 1 teaspoon butter

1   cup chopped pecans

⅓   cup light brown sugar

1   teaspoon vanilla extract

2   cups old-fashioned oats

¼   cup unsweetened coconut flakes

½   cup sunflower seeds

VARIATIONS:

Cinnamon Raisin Granola: Add 1 teaspoon ground cinnamon to brown sugar while cooking. Add raisins after baking.

Almond Cashew Crunch Granola: Use slivered almonds and cashews instead of chopped pecans. Add ½ teaspoon ground cinnamon and ¼ teaspoon ground nutmeg to brown sugar while cooking. Add dried cranberries after baking.

Trail Mix Granola: Use slivered almonds instead of chopped pecans and add raisins and dried apricots after granola has baked.

Sunrise Granola

MAKES 8 SERVINGS • SERVING SIZE: ½ CUP

Homemade granola tastes much better than store-bought versions. It's a good first recipe for kids to make. And, it is hard to make a bad batch, unless you burn it. Nuts burn easily, so keep an eye on them as you toast them.

DIRECTIONS:

Preheat oven to 325 degrees F.

Prepare baking sheet with nonstick spray or line with parchment paper.

In a small saucepan, melt butter over low heat. Add chopped pecans and increase heat to medium, stirring often for 5 minutes or until pecans are lightly toasted. Add brown sugar, reduce heat to low and stir until melted. Remove from heat and stir in vanilla extract.

In a large bowl, combine oats, coconut and sunflower seeds. Add sugar mixture and toss until oats are evenly coated.

Spread granola evenly on prepared cookie sheet. Place in oven on middle rack and bake for 15 minutes. Remove from oven and stir. Bake for another 6 minutes or until golden brown.

Cool completely on baking sheet. Store granola in an airtight container.

 Kid Friendly: Let kids pick the ingredients and name their granola. This boosts their confidence and makes them more likely to eat this healthy cereal.

Less Mess: Plunge the dirty saucepan into soapy water to soak immediately after you pour the sugar mixture into a bowl. Soaking will loosen the sugar mixture.

 Family Time Around the Table: Share your plans for the day.

Love Those Leftovers: Here's a simple way to turn this breakfast cereal into a healthy frozen treat. Roll a banana in peanut butter and then in granola. Put a wooden popsicle stick in the middle, wrap the banana in parchment paper and freeze overnight.

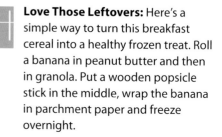 **Nice Price:** Buy nuts on sale and store them in the freezer to preserve freshness.

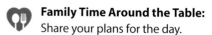

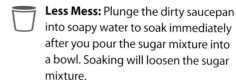

"My 13-year-old and 15-year-old, they're good at breakfast. We do breakfast together. Somebody might do the pancakes. Somebody might do the eggs and somebody else will do the bacon."

NUTRITION FACTS PER SERVING: 290 calories, 20g total fat, 4.5g saturated fat, 10mg cholesterol, 50mg sodium, 26g carbohydrate, 4g dietary fiber, 10g sugar, 9g added sugar, 5g protein

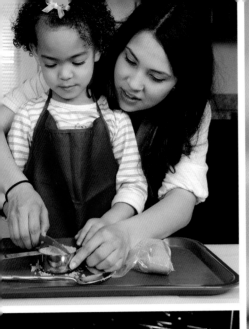

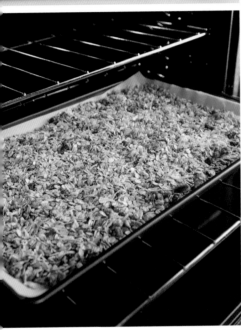

peanut butter,
granola &
banana
pop

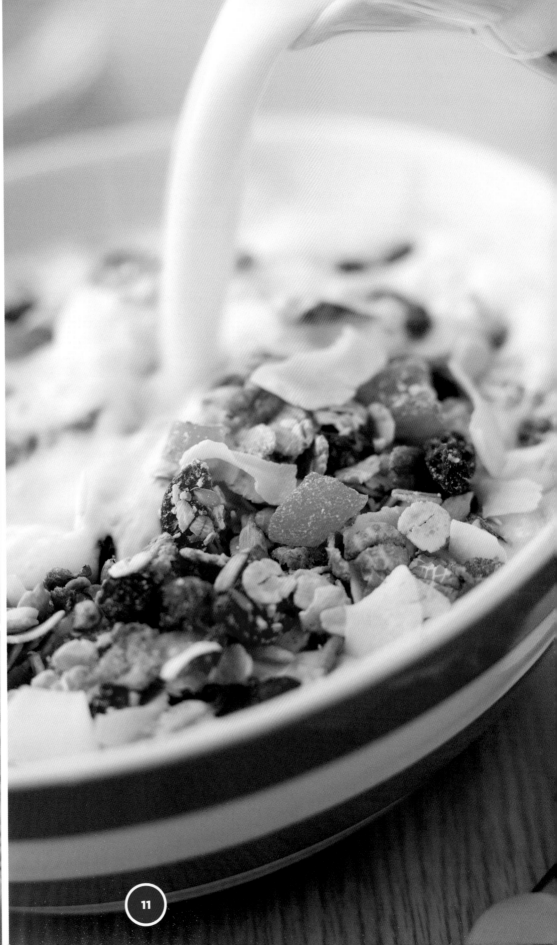

INGREDIENTS:

Nonstick spray or oil

6   eggs

2-3 cups chopped greens or other vegetables

⅓   cup grated Parmesan cheese (1 ounce)

½   teaspoon garlic powder

¼   teaspoon salt

¼   teaspoon ground black pepper

Dash of hot sauce

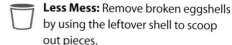

Frittata

MAKES 4 SERVINGS • SERVING SIZE: ¼ OF FRITTATA OR 2 MINI MUFFINS

A frittata is a super-simple Italian omelet that requires no fuss. Whip up some eggs, add some seasoning, pour it in a pan and bake for 10 minutes. You can serve a frittata plain or add your favorite veggies. This dish is good for breakfast, lunch or dinner, and it was a big hit with taste testers.

DIRECTIONS:

Preheat oven to 400 degrees F.

Coat 8-inch round pan or muffin tin (mini frittatas) with nonstick spray or oil, covering bottom and sides. A paper towel can be used to coat pan with oil.

In a medium size bowl whisk eggs until whites and yolks are one color.

Add chopped greens and/or other vegetables. Add cheese, garlic powder, salt and pepper. Mix thoroughly.

Pour egg mixture into prepared pan or muffin tins, three-fourths full.

Bake 10-12 minutes or until eggs are set and an inserted knife comes out clean.

Add a dash of hot sauce to your liking.

 Kid Friendly: Have the kids whip up eggs using a whisk or a fork. This is a fun way to use their boundless energy and to show them how adding air to a mixture changes it.

Less Mess: Remove broken eggshells by using the leftover shell to scoop out pieces.

Family Time Around the Table: Give one compliment to a family member.

Love Those Leftovers: Store your leftover frittata in the refrigerator. Eat cold or reheat in the microwave or under the broiler.

Nice Price: Keep food waste to an absolute minimum by planning your menus.

"My daughter wants to have eggs every day so she can crack them. She does a better job than I do. She doesn't get any shells in the bowl and the yolks are never broken. She does really well for a five-year-old."

NUTRITION FACTS PER SERVING: 140 calories, 9g total fat, 4g saturated fat, 260mg cholesterol, 380mg sodium, 2g carbohydrate, 1g dietary fiber, 0g sugar, 11g protein

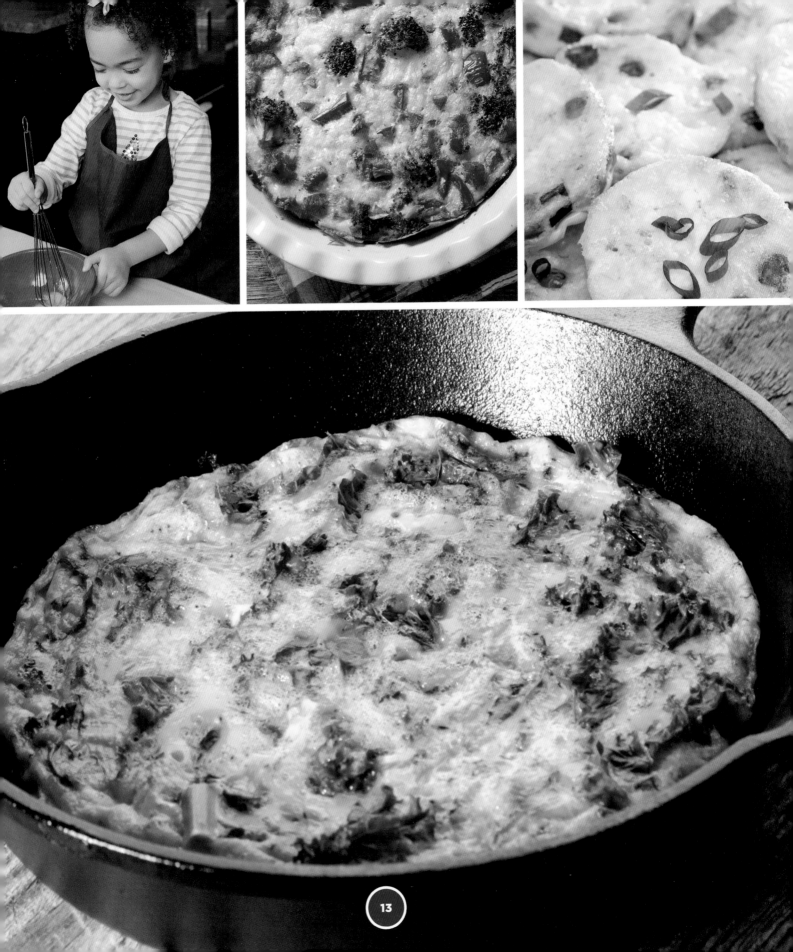

INGREDIENTS:

1 package (10 ounces) chopped, frozen spinach

Nonstick spray or oil

4 eggs

2 cups leftover cooked rice, preferably brown

Salt, pepper and hot sauce to your liking

TOPPINGS (optional):

Shredded cheese, chopped onion, salsa

VARIATIONS:

Hello Again Egg Bowl: Layer bowl with leftover home fries or pasta, vegetables and top with cooked egg.

Buenos Dias Egg Bowl: Layer bowl with leftover meat, rice, salsa and top with cooked egg.

Spinach Rice Egg Bowl

MAKES 4 SERVINGS • SERVING SIZE: 1 EGG BOWL

Cereal isn't the only breakfast food that can be served in a bowl. These warm and nourishing bowls make good use of leftovers and control portion size. Use these recipes as guides, and then tailor them to your tastes and to what's available in your refrigerator and pantry.

DIRECTIONS:

Cook frozen spinach according to package instructions.

Heat nonstick spray or oil in large skillet over medium-high heat.

Fry eggs in skillet until whites are set. Flip and cook one additional minute on reverse side. (More or less, depending on how you like your fried eggs.)

Place rice in a covered saucepan over low heat and sprinkle with water. Stir gently until heated. (Or place rice in microwavable bowl, covered by a wet paper towel, and microwave for 2 minutes.)

Combine rice and spinach in large bowl. Sprinkle with salt, pepper and hot sauce and toss until everything is well distributed.

Divide rice and spinach mixture into 4 bowls. Add one egg to each bowl. Add toppings for additional flavor.

 Kid Friendly: Remind kids to set out spoons, bowls and glasses the night before. Assigning breakfast duties teaches them organizational skills.

 Less Mess: Wear an apron or old button-down shirt to protect clothes.

 Family Time Around the Table: Create morning checklists. Use pictures for younger kids. Morning routines can help everyone get out the door quicker and with less hassle.

 Love Those Leftovers: Store the leftover spinach-rice mixture in the refrigerator. Reheat in the microwave covered with a damp paper towel. Make fried eggs fresh each day to top off your rice bowls.

 Nice Price: Simple recipes that use just a few ingredients not only save money but are often healthier and just as delicious.

"My little boy loves to make scrambled eggs. He wants to help with everything, but breakfast food is his favorite."

NUTRITION FACTS PER SERVING: 190 calories, 5g total fat, 1.5g saturated fat, 165mg cholesterol, 115mg sodium, 26g carbohydrate, 4g dietary fiber, 0g sugar, 10g protein

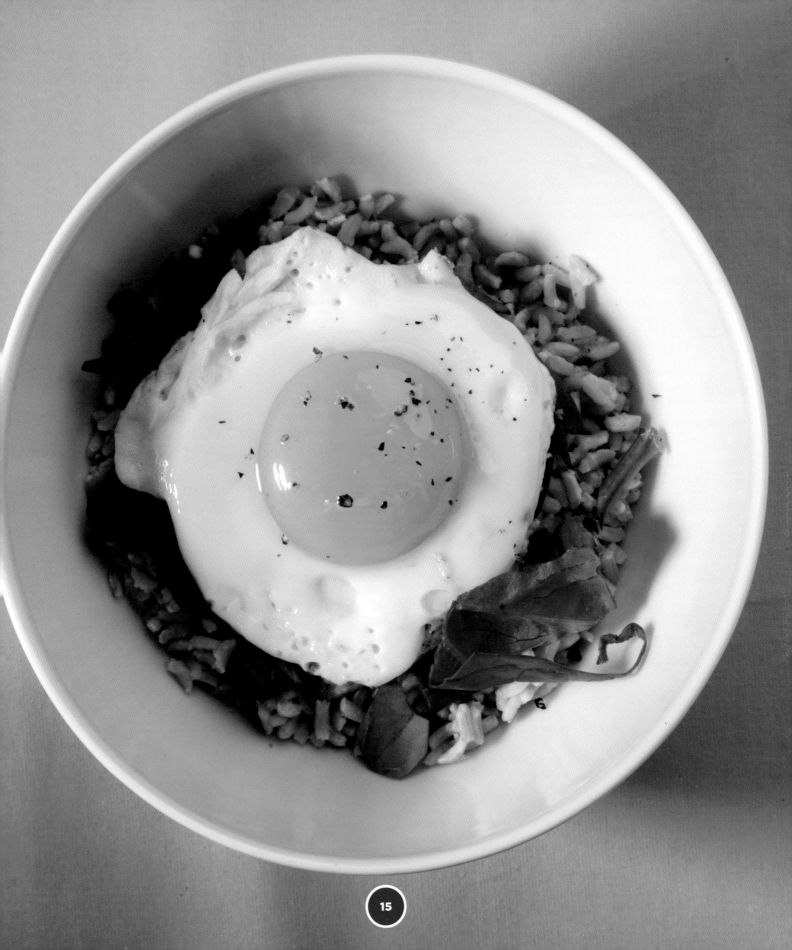

INGREDIENTS:

Nonstick spray or oil

1 cup frozen potatoes with peppers and onions

6 eggs

Salt, pepper and hot sauce to your liking

4 (10-inch) whole wheat tortillas

½ cup shredded cheddar cheese (2 ounces)

Breakfast Burritos

MAKES 4 SERVINGS • SERVING SIZE: 1 BURRITO

Move over fast-food restaurants. Making breakfast burritos at home is cheaper, faster and much tastier. You can even cook breakfast burritos in bulk and freeze them. Homemade breakfast burritos are a healthier start to your day and eliminate the time, trouble and expense of the fast-food drive-thru.

VARIATIONS:

Mexican Breakfast Burritos: Add browned breakfast sausage, Mexican-style chorizo or vegetarian soysage. Add finely shredded Mexican cheese and any or all of the following: salsa, avocado, cilantro, hot sauce and lime.

 TIP Use taco leftovers to make these burritos.

Italian Breakfast Burritos: Add chopped spinach, chopped tomatoes, chopped basil and minced garlic sautéed in olive oil. Add finely shredded mozzarella cheese. Add any or all of the following: grated Parmesan cheese, black olives and hot red pepper flakes.

DIRECTIONS:

In a large skillet heat nonstick spray or oil over medium-high heat.

Add frozen potatoes to skillet and cook, stirring occasionally. Cook until potatoes are golden brown and crisp, 8 to 10 minutes.

Lightly beat eggs in a bowl. Sprinkle with salt and pepper and a couple dashes of hot sauce, if you like. Pour eggs over potatoes and cook, stirring until eggs are fluffy and just set, about 3 minutes.

Remove from skillet and keep warm. Wipe out skillet and return to heat.

Warm tortillas one at a time in the skillet or cover them with wet paper towel and microwave for 30 seconds.

Build burrito by putting egg and potato mixture on the tortilla. Top with cheese. Fold in sides of tortilla and roll up.

 Kid Friendly: Show your kids how to fill, then fold and roll burritos. Involving kids in meal preparation teaches them to be self-sufficient.

 Less Mess: Put ingredients on the tortilla lengthwise. The burrito will roll tighter and less filling will fall out.

 Family Time Around the Table: Name one thing you are looking forward to today.

 Love Those Leftovers: Make extra burritos, wrap individually with parchment paper, place all burritos in one freezer bag and freeze. In the morning, leave the burrito in its paper wrapper and microwave for 30 seconds. Turn burrito over and heat for another 30 seconds.

 Nice Price: Check your local discount store for cheaper parchment paper, foil and plastic wrap.

"When you eat fast-food, in the next hour or two you're back hungry. But when you eat home-cooked food, it seems like you're full longer."

NUTRITION FACTS PER SERVING: 350 calories, 12g total fat, 3.5g saturated fat, 250mg cholesterol, 750mg sodium, 40g carbohydrate, 22g dietary fiber, 1g sugar, 21g protein

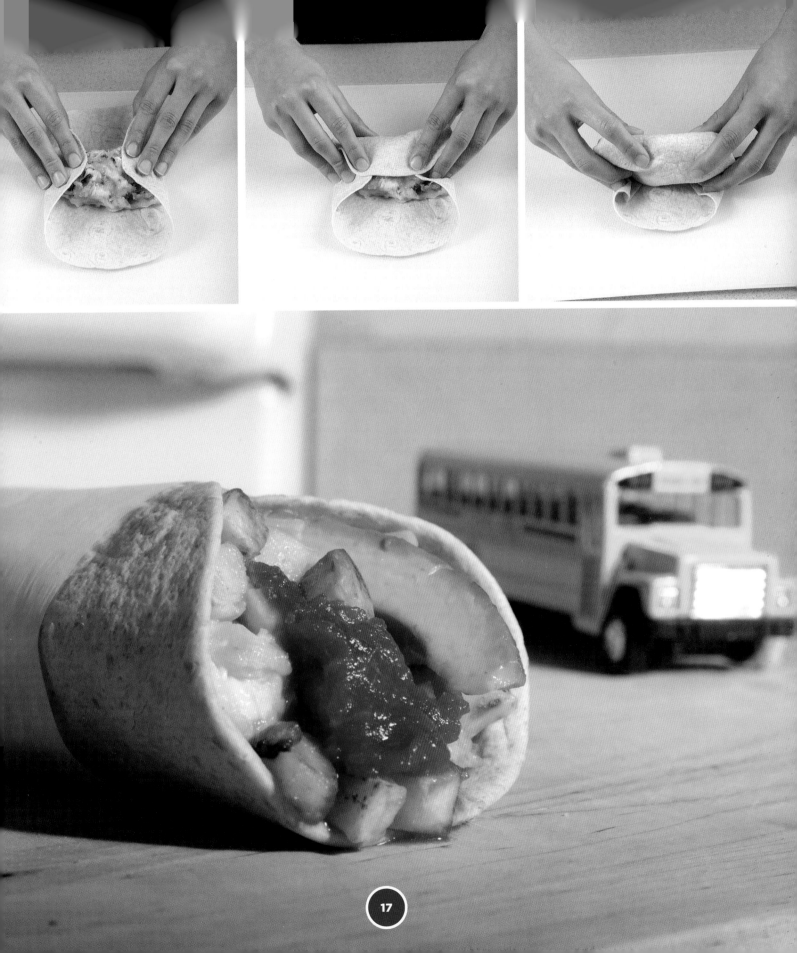

Grab & Go Breakfast

Busy mornings call for quick breakfast solutions. These handheld meals require no preparation or can be fixed quickly and ahead of time. They are all portable and can be eaten in the car, on the bus or as you walk.

trail mix

peanut butter on whole-wheat bread

fruit

hard-boiled egg

yogurt

granola bar

Soups

The aroma of a fragrant soup can melt away the tensions of your day. Soup is fairly simple to make, and you can create your own versions with ingredients you have in your refrigerator and pantry. All you need to get started is broth, vegetables and seasonings. Use the recipes we offer here to learn how to make delicious soups—testers said they were the best soups ever. Or invent your own soup using suggestions in *Making Soup: Your Way*. Soups are a great way to include kids in the cooking process because the recipes are so flexible. Double recipes so you'll have leftovers. The flavors will blend and your soup will be even tastier the next day. Better yet, freeze it for a busy day.

Secrets to Good Soup

◆ To release flavor, give dried herbs a pinch before adding them to the broth.

◆ If soup tastes bland, add a splash of red wine vinegar or lemon juice to brighten the flavor.

◆ A dash of hot sauce can bump up the flavor.

◆ If you're not a vegetarian, use chicken or beef stock to boost flavor.

◆ Make your own broth by simmering leftover vegetables and straining them. You can also use bouillon cubes.

◆ Simmer by cooking gently, just below the boiling point.

◆ Cut vegetables in similar sizes so they cook evenly.

◆ Add vegetables that don't take long to cook—spinach, peppers, corn—later in the process so they don't get mushy.

◆ Create a toppings bar so everyone can fix their bowl as they like it. Some ideas for your bar: fresh herbs like cilantro and/or parsley, Greek yogurt or sour cream, lemon or lime wedges, salsa, shredded cheese or Parmesan, crumbled bacon and green onions.

◆ Add alphabet pasta to make dinner more fun and to stimulate conversation. Are there any words in your spoon?

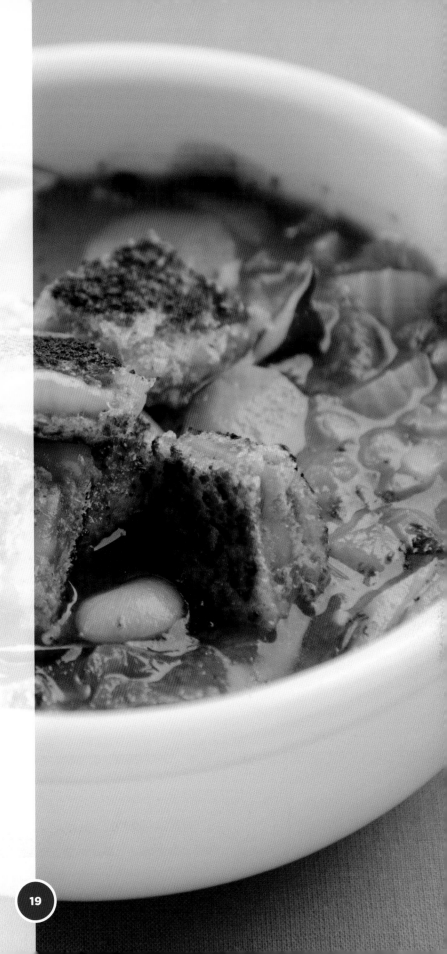

INGREDIENTS:

- 1 tablespoon butter
- 1 tablespoon olive oil
- 1 medium yellow onion, chopped
- 2 stalks celery, chopped
- 2 medium carrots, peeled and chopped
- 2 medium yellow (Yukon) potatoes, chopped, peeled or unpeeled
- 2 teaspoons garlic, minced or 1 teaspoon garlic powder
- 2 quarts canned or boxed low-sodium vegetable broth
- 1 small zucchini, chopped
- ¼ cup green or purple cabbage, coarsely chopped
- 1 ear of corn, cut off the cob or 1 cup frozen or canned yellow sweet corn, drained and rinsed
- 1 package (12 ounces) frozen baby lima beans or 1 can (15 ounces) baby lima beans, drained and rinsed
- 1 package (28 ounces) frozen mixed vegetables or 2 cans (11 ounces) mixed vegetables, drained and rinsed
- 1 can (28 ounces) diced tomatoes, with liquid
- 2 teaspoons Italian seasoning
- 2 bay leaves
  Salt and pepper to your liking
  Dash of hot sauce, optional

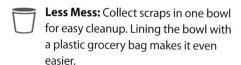

Hearty Vegetable Soup

MAKES 12 SERVINGS • SERVING SIZE: 1½ CUPS

Moms from across Kentucky were quick to name vegetable soup as one of their favorite meals. All agreed that learning to make a good pot of vegetable soup is a skill worth having. This recipe is a good start, but keep in mind you can change it based on the veggies and other ingredients that you have on hand. The great thing about vegetable soup is that it isn't picky. Use fresh or frozen vegetables or a combination of both. Try grilled cheese croutons for a fun change. You can make grilled cheese croutons by cutting a basic grilled cheese sandwich into 1-inch squares.

DIRECTIONS:

In a large soup pot, sauté onions, celery, carrots, potatoes and garlic in melted butter and olive oil over medium-low heat about 5 minutes or until tender.

Add broth and remaining vegetables, including can of tomatoes with liquid.

Add Italian seasoning and bay leaves. Bring to gentle boil, then lower heat to simmer.

Simmer about 15 minutes or until carrots and potatoes are tender. Remove bay leaves before serving.

Add salt and pepper to your liking. Keep in mind that store-bought broth has added salt.

TIP Don't forget to add a dash of hot sauce if you like a little kick!

 Kid Friendly: Show older kids how to cut vegetables using safe knife skills. This helps them learn the basics of kitchen safety.

 Less Mess: Collect scraps in one bowl for easy cleanup. Lining the bowl with a plastic grocery bag makes it even easier.

 Family Time Around the Table: Share your favorite part or biggest challenge of the day.

Love Those Leftovers: Freeze soup in muffin tins for single portions that reheat quickly. Freeze the portions, place them in a plastic freezer bag and store in the freezer for up to three months.

 Nice Price: When in season, shop for ingredients at the local farmers' market. Be flexible and buy larger quantities when it is affordable. Farmers will often make a deal when customers buy in bulk.

"Homemade vegetable soup, now that's my main vegetable."

NUTRITION FACTS PER SERVING: 150 calories, 2.5g total fat, 1g saturated fat, 5mg cholesterol, 310mg sodium, 25g carbohydrate, 6g dietary fiber, 7g sugar, 7g protein

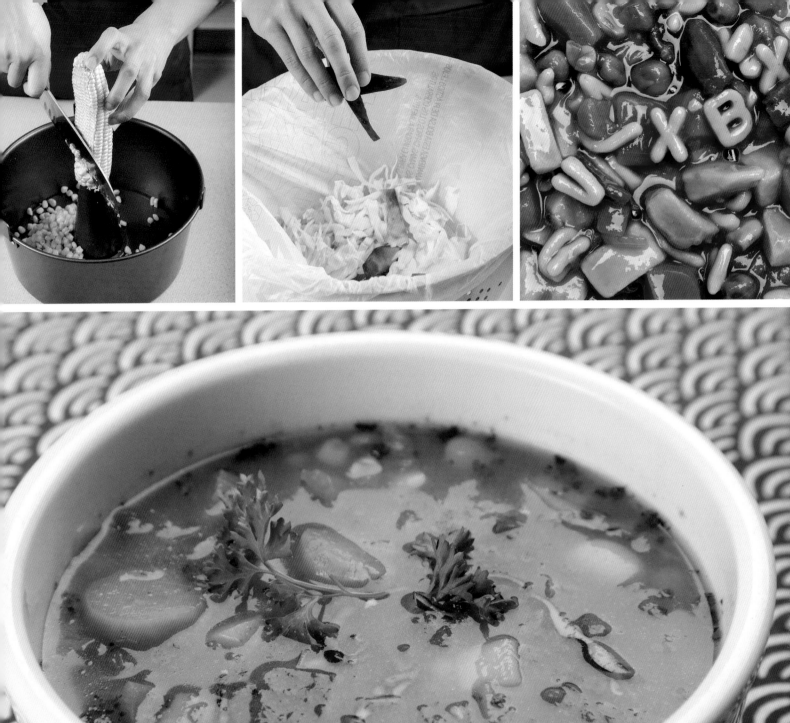

INGREDIENTS:

- 1 tablespoon butter
- 1 tablespoon olive oil
- 1 medium yellow onion, chopped
- 3 cloves garlic, minced or 1 tablespoon garlic powder
- 2 cups red potatoes, peeled and chopped
- ½ cup carrots, peeled and shredded
- 2 cups fresh broccoli, chopped or 1 package (10 ounces) frozen broccoli florets
- 3½ tablespoons all-purpose flour
- 4 cups fat-free, low-sodium chicken broth (or vegetable broth or vegetarian no-chicken broth)
- 1 cup half-and-half
- ¼ teaspoon ground nutmeg
- 1 cup shredded low-fat cheddar cheese (4 ounces)

  Salt and pepper to your liking

Creamy Broccoli Soup

MAKES 8 SERVINGS • SERVING SIZE: 1½ CUP

This recipe takes the flavor of the beloved broccoli casserole and turns it into a lower fat, lower calorie soup that is far better than any canned versions. Add garlic butter croutons for more flavor and crunch. To make the croutons, cut stale bread into small cubes, toss with a small amount of melted butter and garlic powder and broil the bread until it is golden brown. Watch closely because the croutons burn easily.

DIRECTIONS:

In a large soup pot, sauté onions and garlic in melted butter and oil over medium-high heat about 2 minutes or until tender. Add potatoes, carrots and broccoli one at a time and sauté each about 2 minutes. Stir in flour and toss until vegetables are coated. Cook 1-2 minutes.

Gradually add broth, stirring constantly. Bring to a boil.

Reduce heat to low and simmer covered for 25 minutes.

Remove lid and stir in half-and-half slowly. Simmer uncovered for 20 minutes, stirring occasionally. Do not boil. For thicker soup, blend 2 cups of broth with vegetables and return the mixture to soup.

Add nutmeg.

Add cheese and let melt. Stir gently. Add salt and pepper to your liking. Serve.

Kid Friendly: Allow older kids to shred the carrots and cheese. Remind them that tools like the shredder are sharp and can cut them.

Less Mess: Clean the kitchen while the soup simmers. Cleaning as you go makes things easier.

Family Time Around the Table: Describe the most beautiful place you have ever seen.

Love Those Leftovers: Make an easy chicken, rice and broccoli casserole. In a bowl, combine cooked chicken pieces and cooked rice with the leftover Creamy Broccoli Soup. Spray a casserole dish with nonstick spray and spread the mixture in it. Bake covered with foil at 350 degrees F for 30 minutes. Remove foil and bake another 10 minutes.

Nice Price: Buy cheese by the block and shred it yourself. Look for an inexpensive cheese grater at a discount or dollar store.

"At supper time at my house, there are no phones, no TV, no computer. It's time to talk about what happened at school. What did you learn? What did you do?"

NUTRITION FACTS PER SERVING: 220 calories, 11g total fat, 5g saturated fat, 20mg cholesterol, 630mg sodium, 20g carbohydrate, 2g dietary fiber, 1g sugar, 8 g protein

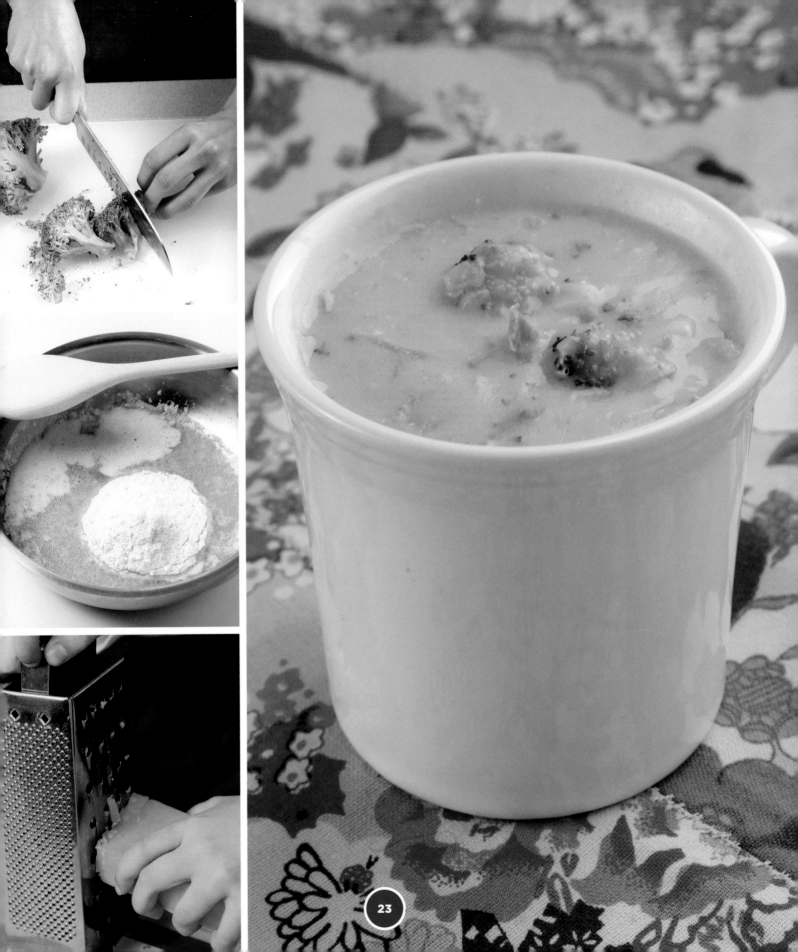

INGREDIENTS:

- 2 tablespoons olive oil
- 1 medium yellow onion, chopped
- 2 stalks celery, chopped (including some leaves)
- 4 medium carrots, peeled and chopped
- 2 quarts fat-free, low-sodium chicken broth
- 2 cups chicken breast, cooked and shredded
- ½ teaspoon whole black peppercorns
- 2 teaspoons dried thyme leaves
- 2 bay leaves
- 2 cups all-purpose flour
- 2 teaspoons baking powder
- ¾ cup low-fat milk
- 1 egg
- 2 cups coarsely chopped fresh kale leaves (Any greens can be used.)

Chicken and Dumpling Soup

MAKES 10 SERVINGS • SERVING SIZE: 2 CUPS

Kentucky mothers agree that chicken and dumplings are the essence of good home cooking. This soup has chicken and tender dumplings with savory vegetables in a warm, flavorful broth. Dumplings are easier to make than you might think. Make a simple dough, roll it and cut the dough into flat strips or drop it into the soup by the spoonful.

DIRECTIONS:

In a large soup pot, sauté onions, celery and carrots in olive oil over medium-low heat for about 5 minutes or until tender.

Add broth, chicken, peppercorns, thyme and bay leaves. Reduce heat to low. Simmer partially covered for 20 minutes.

Meanwhile, in a small bowl, mix flour, baking powder, milk and egg until well blended. Roll out with a rolling pin and make strips or simply drop small spoonfuls of dough into simmering soup.

Cover soup and allow dumplings to cook about 20 minutes. They will rise to the top of the soup as they cook.

Stir in kale, cover soup and simmer 5 additional minutes. Remove bay leaves and peppercorns before serving soup.

TIP If you'd rather not make dumplings, add egg noodles 8 minutes before serving.

 Kid Friendly: Let the kids prepare the dumplings. Warn them not to stir the dough too much; it will not rise if it has been over stirred.

 Less Mess: Put plastic wrap directly on counter, place dough on top and then put another layer over the dough before rolling it out to keep countertops and rolling pins clean.

 Family Time Around the Table: Discuss an interesting current event. For small children, this might be what happened to the neighbor's cat today. For older children, it can be a story in the news.

 Love Those Leftovers: Store leftover soup in the refrigerator. The soup will be even better the next day. Reheat gently. You may need to add a little more broth or water.

 Nice Price: Roast a chicken for this recipe and use the leftover carcass, bones and veggies to make an easy broth that freezes well.

"We use cooking as a major educational tool at our house. It's the best. My daughter loves to mix. I will measure out the ingredients and set them on the counter and she will just dump them together."

NUTRITION FACTS PER SERVING: 200 calories, 4.5g total fat, 1g saturated fat, 40mg cholesterol, 540mg sodium, 24g carbohydrate, 2g dietary fiber, 3g sugar, 15g protein

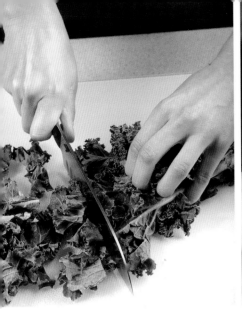
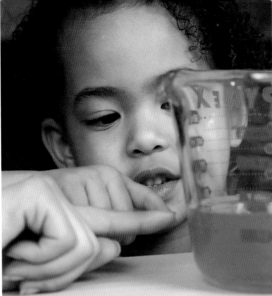
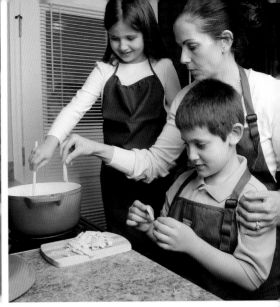
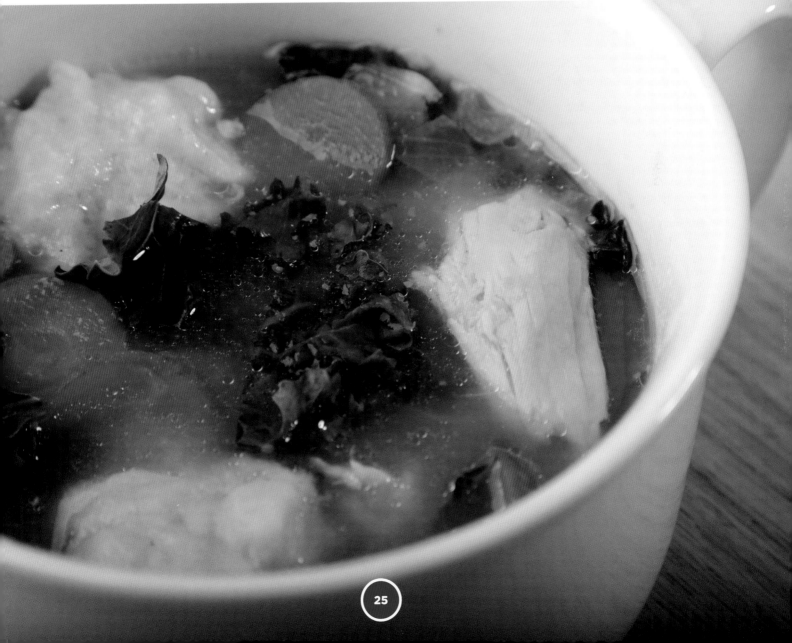

Making Soup: Your Way

Making soup is a great way to use leftover vegetables and meats. You don't even need a recipe. Follow these simple steps and make a delicious soup from whatever you have on hand. Give the soup you create a name and turn it into a family tradition and a mealtime favorite.

Basics for Making Soup

◆ In a large pot over medium-high heat, sauté aromatic vegetables (onion, carrots, celery, garlic) with butter or olive oil.

◆ If you are using meat, cook it separately.

◆ Add about 4 cups of any base you already have: chicken, beef or shellfish stock, vegetable broth, tomato purée or even water.

◆ Add vegetables that need a longer time to cook first: potatoes, sweet potatoes, carrots and winter squash.

◆ Add dried beans that have been soaked overnight or have had a quick soak. For a quick soak, rinse the beans in a colander with cool running water, transfer to pot, cover with clean water, and bring to a boil. Take off heat and let beans soak in the hot water for about an hour.

◆ Add cooked meat.

◆ Add dried seasonings: thyme leaves, parsley leaves, celery seed, garlic powder, basil leaves, oregano leaves, rosemary leaves, bay leaves and/or mint leaves.

◆ Bring soup to a boil, lower heat and cover pot with lid. Let simmer at least 1 hour.

◆ Add pasta or cooked rice if desired.

◆ Add milk or cream if desired.

◆ Taste and adjust. Add extra flavor with lemon juice, vinegar, hot sauce and/or ground pepper.

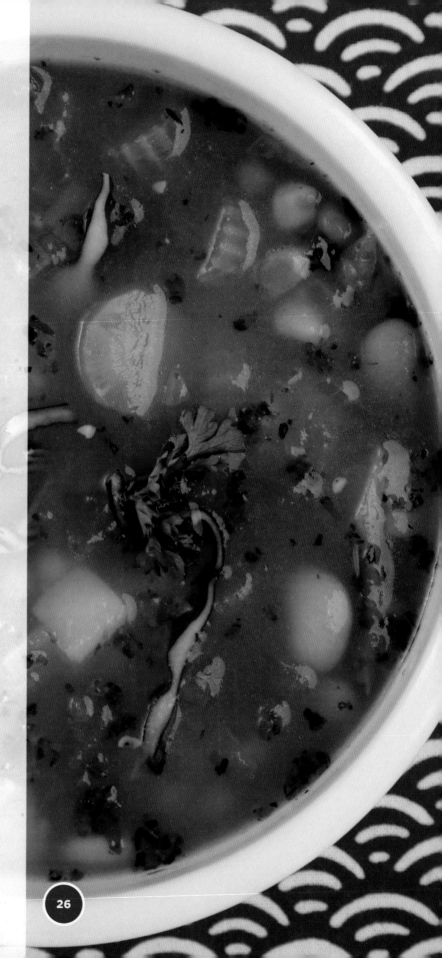

Salads

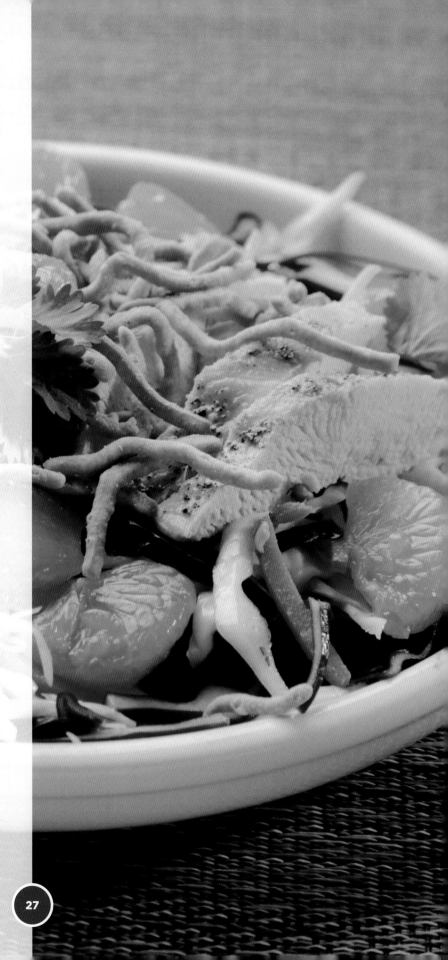

It's hard to go wrong with a salad. All you need is a few fresh vegetables, some flavorful add-ins and a splash of something tangy like lemon juice or vinegar. Try seasonal fruits and vegetables that you've bought at the store, produce stand, farmers' market or that you've harvested from your garden.

How to Make a Great Salad on a Budget

◆ **Small Portions.** Salads don't have to be huge. They can simply be a little something fresh on the side to perk up a meal.

◆ **Create a Dinner Salad.** To turn a salad into a meal, combine any of the following on top of a bed of lettuce: a can of tuna; chopped, hard-boiled eggs; sunflower seeds; leftover rice or pasta; shredded cheese; drained, canned chickpeas; leftover cooked broccoli. Or set up a salad bar and let your family create their own salad.

◆ **Dry Thoroughly.** Nobody likes soggy lettuce. Wash and dry it thoroughly using one of three methods: (1) Wash lettuce in a colander. Put it in a clean pillowcase that you use only for the kitchen. (Have the kids write 'Kitchen' on it.) Close the pillowcase opening with your hand and swing it around until the water spins out. This is a perfect job for kids. (2) Rinse, drain and blot lettuce on a clean dish towel or a couple of paper towels. (3) Salad spinners work well and are a great investment when they can be purchased on sale.

◆ **Use Vegetables at Their Freshest.** Use the freshest vegetables—those that have been in the fridge a day or two—to make a salad. Save veggies that aren't as fresh for soups and other cooked dishes.

◆ **Fresh and Crisp.** Take a tip from nice restaurants and chill salad bowls or plates. It's a little touch that makes salads taste fresher and crisper.

◆ **Well Dressed.** You can always add more dressing to a salad, but you can't undress a salad so add just a little at a time. To make homemade dressings, use the recipes we offer here or use the information in *Making Salad Dressings: Your Way* to invent your own.

INGREDIENTS:

DRESSING:

- 2 tablespoons olive oil
- 2 tablespoons honey (or brown sugar)
- 2 tablespoons apple cider vinegar
- ½ lime, juiced (about 1 tablespoon)
  Salt and pepper to your liking

SALAD:

- 2 cups green cabbage, shredded
- 2 cups purple cabbage, shredded
- 1 Granny Smith apple, chopped
- 2 medium carrots, peeled and shredded
- 2 stalks celery, chopped
- ½ small red onion, chopped
- ⅓ cup sunflower seeds
- ⅓ cup raisins
  Small handful of chopped cilantro and/or parsley, optional

Crunchy Apple & Cabbage Salad

MAKES 10 SERVINGS • SERVING SIZE: 1 CUP

Cabbage is an excellent food bargain. A head of cabbage chopped in small pieces will fill a huge bowl. This recipe has big flavor and crunch. It also provides an opportunity to channel your inner celebrity chef and perfect your chopping skills. The better you become at chopping, the more you will enjoy cooking.

DIRECTIONS:

Whisk olive oil and remaining dressing ingredients in the bottom of a large bowl.

Add cabbage and remaining salad ingredients to bowl with dressing. Toss well until salad is evenly coated. If preparing ahead of time, chop and add the apple right before serving so the apple pieces don't brown.

 Kid Friendly: Help kids measure raisins and sunflower seeds. Learning basic skills like measuring is always useful.

 Less Mess: Make dressing in the bottom of a large container, and then add salad ingredients. Toss salad and dressing without dirtying another dish.

 Family Time Around the Table: Name one thing you are grateful for today.

 Love Those Leftovers: Add grilled chicken for a simple, healthy lunch. Add mandarin oranges and crispy chow mein noodles for an Asian twist.

 Nice Price: Buy cabbage by the head and shred it instead of buying prepackaged, shredded cabbage. One head of cabbage can be used for several recipes.

"I mean just look at your kids.
Really, honestly, you want to live as long as you can…"

NUTRITION FACTS PER SERVING: 120 calories, 5g total fat, 0.5g saturated fat, 0mg cholesterol, 55mg sodium, 16g carbohydrate, 3g dietary fiber, 11g sugar, 2g protein

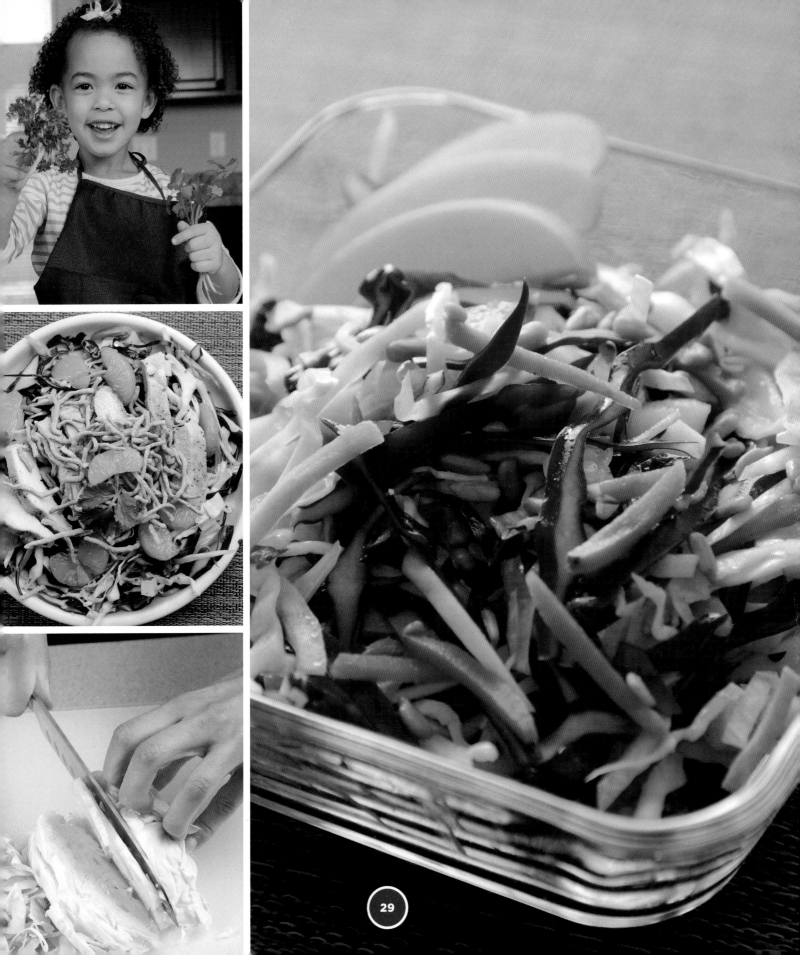

Southern Cornbread Salad

INGREDIENTS:

1 package (8.5 ounces) corn muffin mix

DRESSING:

1 cup plain Greek or regular yogurt

2 teaspoons low-fat mayonnaise

2 teaspoons all-purpose seasoning

2 teaspoons dried dill weed

2 teaspoons ground black pepper

1½ teaspoons fresh garlic, minced or
    ½ teaspoon garlic powder

½ teaspoon salt

SALAD:

1 can (15 ounces) light kidney beans,
   drained and rinsed

3 cups frozen yellow sweet corn, thawed
   or 3 cans (15 ounces) no salt added
   whole kernel corn, drained and rinsed

1 small red onion, chopped

1 bell pepper, chopped

2 large tomatoes, chopped

3 slices bacon, crisp-cooked
   and crumbled

1½ cups shredded cheddar cheese
    (6 ounces)

1 bundle green onions, chopped

This layered salad is a meal in a bowl. The flavors and colors complement each other perfectly to make a dish that is beautiful and delicious. This healthier version of a cornbread salad and ranch dressing could make your family's favorites list.

DIRECTIONS:

Bake cornbread according to package directions. Let stand until cool. Cut cornbread into 1-inch cubes.

Mix yogurt, mayonnaise, all-purpose seasoning, dill weed, pepper, garlic and salt in a bowl. Set aside.

In a large bowl layer cornbread, beans, corn, onion, bell peppers, tomatoes and bacon. Spread dressing mixture over salad. Cover with cheese. Top with chopped green onions.

Kid Friendly: Kids can mix the cornbread ingredients. They are more likely to be interested in foods they help prepare.

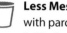

Less Mess: Line skillet or cake pan with parchment paper or aluminum foil before you bake the cornbread.

Family Time Around the Table: Play I-Spy with your meal. Say the first letter of an ingredient and take turns trying to guess its identity.

Love Those Leftovers: Use leftover cornbread for this salad. Use any leftover ranch dressing for tossed salads and veggie dip.

Nice Price: Make your own salad dressings. This recipe for ranch dressing is cheaper than store-bought brands and is much healthier.

"I think for me, I'm a Southerner, I learned all the wrong ways to make everything taste good, you know? So, I think I just want to learn how to make things taste better the natural way, so I could live a lot longer."

NUTRITION FACTS PER SERVING: 240 calories, 9g total fat, 4g saturated fat, 30mg cholesterol, 620mg sodium, 28g carbohydrate, 5g dietary fiber, 8g sugar, 12g protein

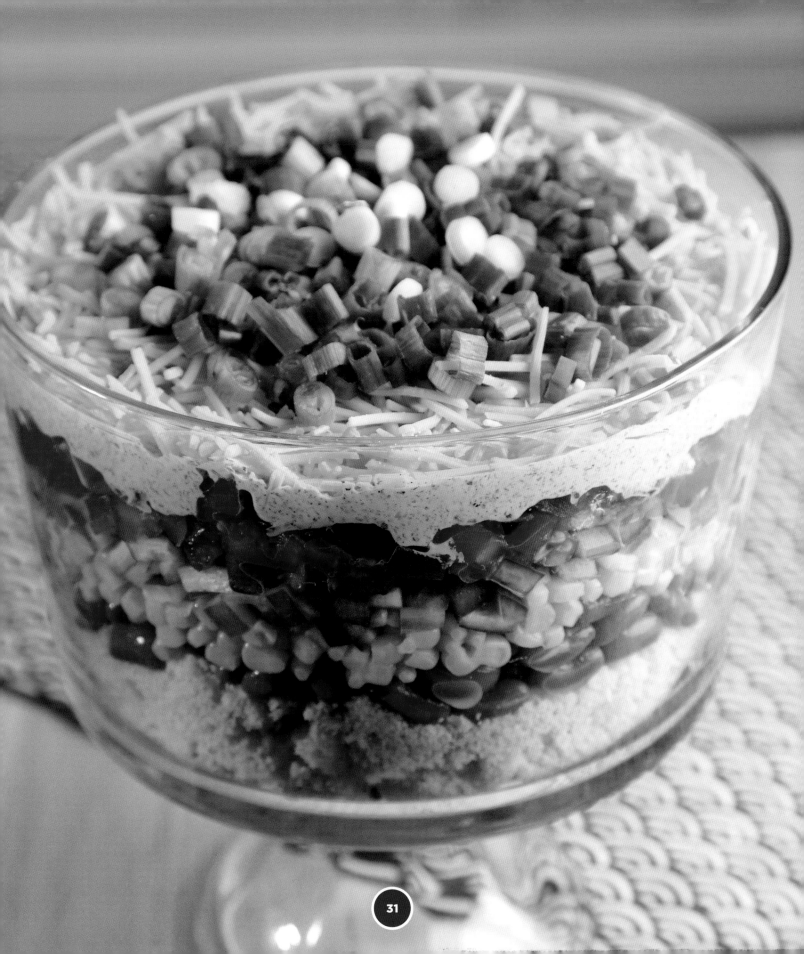

INGREDIENTS:

DRESSING:

- ⅔ cup plain Greek or regular yogurt
- ⅓ cup milk
- 1 teaspoon ground cumin
- 1 teaspoon chili powder
- ½ lime, juiced (about 1 tablespoon)
- Salt to your liking

SALAD:

- 1 head romaine lettuce, torn into bite-size pieces
- 1 tomato, chopped
- ½ small red onion, chopped
- 1 cup frozen sweet yellow corn, thawed or 1 can (15 ounces) no salt added whole-kernel corn, drained and rinsed
- 1 can (15 ounces) black beans, drained and rinsed
- 2 cups shredded roasted chicken, optional
- 1 cup crushed tortilla chips, optional

Fresh Taco Salad

MAKES 10 SERVINGS • SERVING SIZE: 1⅓ CUPS

Many taco salads are so heavy and greasy that they probably shouldn't even be considered a salad. This recipe is light and fresh but still satisfying. The creamy dressing recipe received high marks from taste testers.

DIRECTIONS:

Mix the dressing ingredients in a bowl. Let stand at least 5 minutes.

Combine lettuce, tomato, onion, corn and beans in a large bowl. Add dressing to individual servings. Top with chicken and tortilla chips, if desired.

 Kid Friendly: Let kids take turns 'spin drying' the lettuce. Kids can also help tear lettuce into bite-size pieces. When food preparation is fun, they will be more willing to help out.

 Less Mess: Don't have a salad spinner? Put washed lettuce in a clean, cotton pillowcase or a plastic grocery bag lined with paper towels and spin it around in circles.

 Family Time Around the Table: Television can be a big distraction. Take some time to turn the TV and other electronics off and focus on each other.

 Love Those Leftovers: Turn leftover taco salad into a lunch wrap. Put salad on a whole wheat tortilla, add salad dressing and fold the tortilla.

 Nice Price: Check out spices in the Mexican food aisle. They are often cheaper than the baking section. Store in containers with tight-fitting lids to preserve freshness. Baby food jars work great.

"My mom made sure we knew how to cook. We started helping when we were real young. It's the same way I teach my children. It's important that they know how to cook."

NUTRITION FACTS PER SERVING: 70 calories, 0.5g total fat, 0g saturated fat, 0mg cholesterol, 150mg sodium, 12g carbohydrate, 4g dietary fiber, 3g sugar, 5g protein
IF USING CHICKEN, ADD (PER SERVING): 50 calories, 1g total fat, 0g saturated fat, 25mg cholesterol, 20mg sodium, 0g carbohydrate, 0g dietary fiber, 0g sugar, 9g protein
IF USING TORTILLA CHIPS, ADD (PER SERVING): 30 calories, 1g total fat, 0g saturated fat, 0mg cholesterol, 30mg sodium, 5g carbohydrate, 0g dietary fiber, 0g sugar, 1g protein

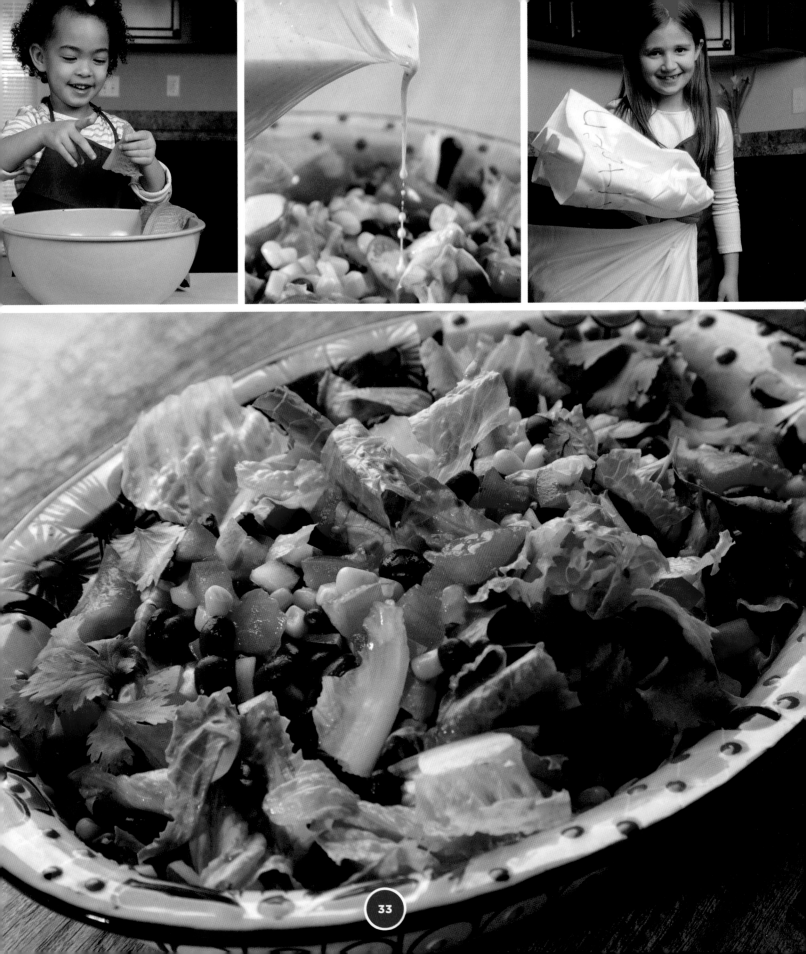

Making Salad Dressings: Your Way

Learning to make good salads will help your kids learn to love vegetables. The dressing for your salad should be as healthy as the salad. You will find that most homemade salad dressings take only a couple of minutes to make, require no specialized equipment and can be fine-tuned to suit any family member's taste buds. An added bonus is that homemade dressings cost a lot less than the store-bought versions. After you try these simple dressing recipes, you may never buy bottled dressing again.

TIP Try serving salads first the way restaurants do. Eating salad first slows you down, ensures that you eat some veggies and fills you up so you may eat less during the rest of the meal.

Homemade Salad Dressing

Whether it is a creamy dressing or a simple vinaigrette, all dressings have 5 basic ingredients:

1. **Oil:** Use olive oil or any neutral-tasting alternative like canola or safflower oil. How much oil do you need? The oil-to-acid ratio for most dressings is 3 to 1. However, you may adjust the ratio to your liking. If creamy dressing is more your family's style, add mayonnaise, milk or buttermilk as your base.

2. **Acid:** The go-to vinegars are balsamic, apple cider, red wine and white wine. You can also substitute some or all of the vinegar with fresh-squeezed lemon or lime juice. A splash of lime juice goes well with citrus-based salads.

3. **Sweet:** To make acid taste less bitter, add a little sugar. White sugar will do, but you'll add more flavor with honey, maple syrup, apple juice, frozen orange juice concentrate or jam.

4. **Salt:** A generous pinch is often enough. You can also season individual servings to make everyone happy.

5. **Aromatics:** Minced fresh herbs, shallots, citrus rind, black pepper and/or garlic add flavor and variety. Popular salad herbs include basil, thyme, tarragon, cilantro, mint, parsley and dill.

To make your dressing, place all ingredients in a small jar with a tight-fitting lid and shake. If you are using a small bowl, whisk the oil into the other ingredients. Store unused dressing in the refrigerator.

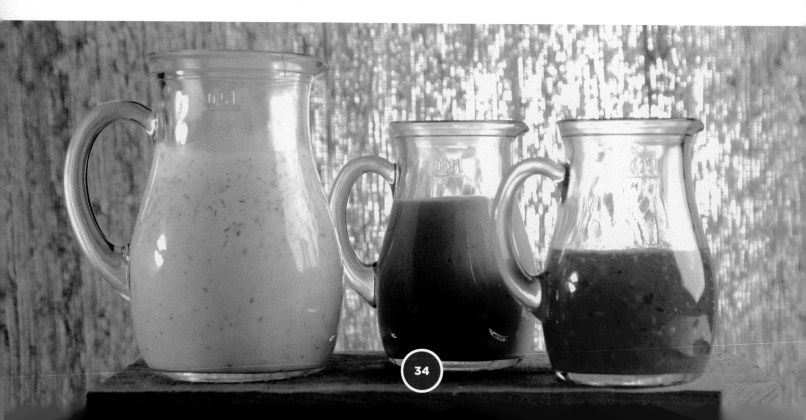

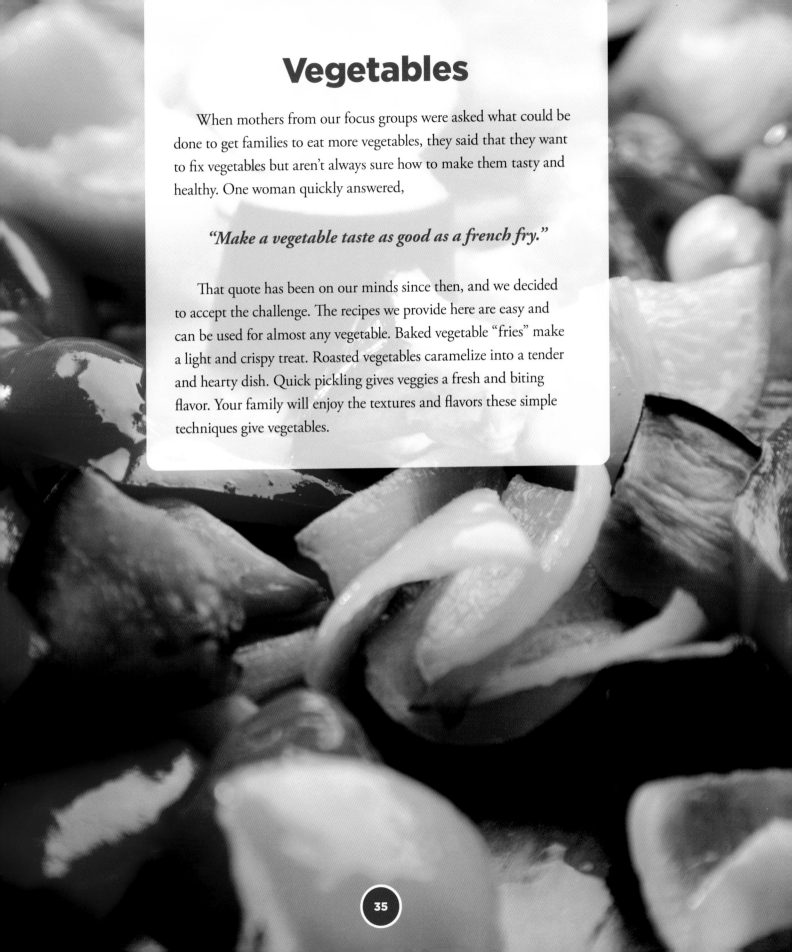

Vegetables

When mothers from our focus groups were asked what could be done to get families to eat more vegetables, they said that they want to fix vegetables but aren't always sure how to make them tasty and healthy. One woman quickly answered,

"Make a vegetable taste as good as a french fry."

That quote has been on our minds since then, and we decided to accept the challenge. The recipes we provide here are easy and can be used for almost any vegetable. Baked vegetable "fries" make a light and crispy treat. Roasted vegetables caramelize into a tender and hearty dish. Quick pickling gives veggies a fresh and biting flavor. Your family will enjoy the textures and flavors these simple techniques give vegetables.

INGREDIENTS:

- ½ cup all-purpose flour
- Pinch of salt
- ½ teaspoon pepper
- 1 egg plus one egg white, beaten
- ½ cup panko bread crumbs
- ¼ cup grated Parmesan cheese (¾ ounce)
- ½ teaspoon paprika
- 4 medium zucchini, sliced ½-inch thick and 4 inches long
- Nonstick spray

VARIATIONS:

- 1 pound bag of parsnips, peeled and cut into strips the shape of fries
- 1 pound bag of carrots, peeled and cut into strips the shape of fries
- 2 large sweet potatoes, peeled and cut into strips the shape of fries
- 2 large avocados peeled and cut into strips the shape of fries (These are popular in trendy restaurants.)

Crispy Oven Zucchini "Fries"

MAKES 8 SERVINGS • SERVING SIZE: 1 CUP

These golden "fries" mimic the crunchy outside and tender inside of regular french fries. After you try this technique, you won't ever deep fry again. Experiment with different vegetables to find your family's favorites.

DIRECTIONS:

Preheat oven to 450 degrees F.

Add flour to a pie plate and whisk in salt and pepper. Beat eggs together in a second pie plate.

In a third pie plate, whisk the panko, Parmesan, paprika and another dash of salt and pepper.

Dip zucchini slices in the flour, then in the egg and then through the breadcrumb mixture. Place on a baking sheet treated with nonstick spray. Bake for 10 minutes, turn slices and continue cooking for another 10 minutes until golden and crisp.

 Kid Friendly: Kids will like dipping veggies into the flour, egg and breadcrumbs. Teach them to wash their hands often to avoid germs.

 Less Mess: Line the baking tray with foil for easy cleanup. Take dirty dishes to the sink as soon as possible.

 Family Time Around the Table: Come up with a family motto.

 Love Those Leftovers: Use leftover homemade ranch dressing or taco salad dressing as a dipping sauce. Or add some spice to your ketchup. Try garlic, basil, curry powder, hot sauce or horseradish.

 Nice Price: Panko is a crunchy breadcrumb made from crustless bread. Save money by using day-old bread you have on hand. Remove crust and crumble. Spread evenly on a baking sheet and bake at 300 degrees F for 4 minutes or just long enough to dry out the crumbs.

"Honey, you have to have vegetables."

NUTRITION FACTS PER SERVING: 90 calories, 2g total fat, 1g saturated fat, 25mg cholesterol, 85mg sodium, 13g carbohydrate, 1g dietary fiber, 2g sugar, 5g protein

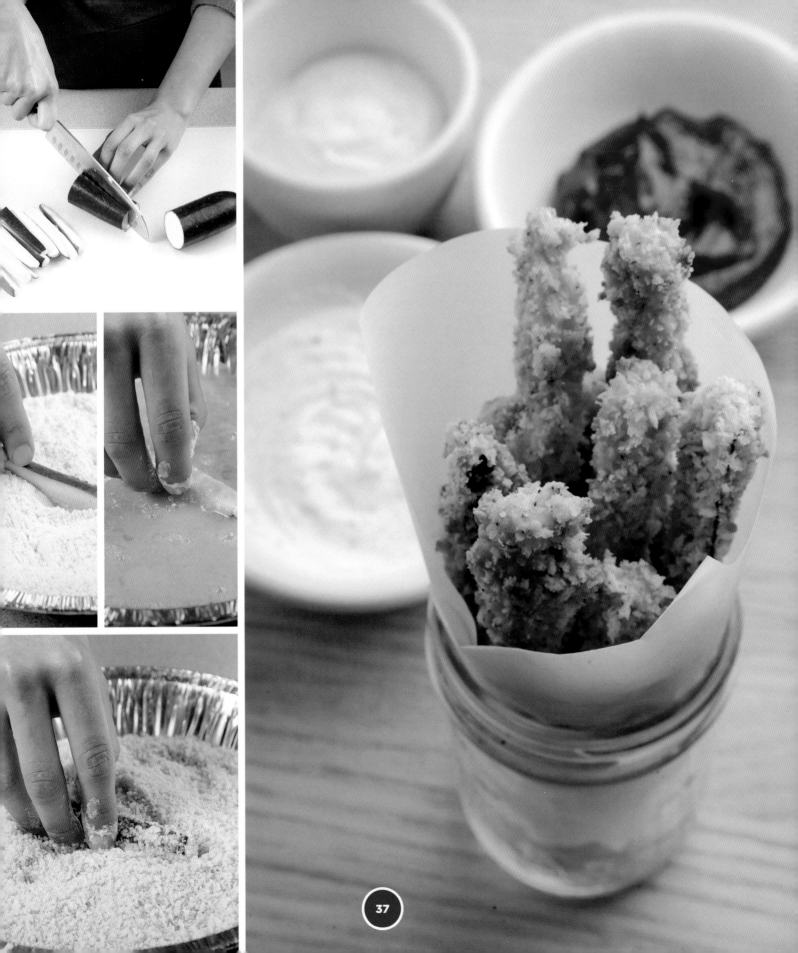

Roasted Vegetables

MAKES 8 SERVINGS • SERVING SIZE: ½ CUP

Roasting vegetables brings out sweet and savory flavors better than any other cooking method. Vegetables become slightly brown, crisp and surprisingly flavorful when they come in contact with the heat of the dry pan during roasting. Use vegetables you have on hand and make this a regular part of your meals.

INGREDIENTS:

- 2 tablespoons olive oil
- 3 pounds assorted vegetables, prepared and cut into bite size pieces (See below for seasonal variations.)
- 4 cloves garlic, whole
- 1 lemon, cut into 1 inch wedges

  Salt and pepper to your liking

VARIATIONS:

Spring: carrots, asparagus, mushrooms, spring onions, radishes and thyme. If you use fresh thyme, discard sprigs before serving.

Summer: yellow onion, red pepper, zucchini, cherry tomatoes, summer squash and eggplant. Sprinkle with fresh or dried basil leaves before serving.

DIRECTIONS:

Preheat oven to 425 degrees F.

Combine vegetables, garlic, lemon and oil in a bowl. Add salt and pepper to your liking. Toss to coat.

Line a baking sheet with foil. Spread vegetables and lemon in a single layer. (If vegetables are stacked, they steam rather than roast and the flavor is not as good. Depending on the amount of vegetables, you might need two pans to ensure all the vegetables are touching the pan.)

Place baking sheet on the middle rack. Roast about 20 minutes or until vegetables are tender, yet firm in the center. Stir halfway through to make sure vegetables don't stick or burn. Discard lemon before serving.

 Kid Friendly: Allow your kids to pick one veggie per shopping trip. Kids are more likely to eat the veggies they choose.

 Less Mess: Place a wet paper towel under your cutting board to keep it from sliding. This improves safety and keeps the counter cleaner.

 Family Time Around the Table: Name a superpower you would like to have and why.

 Love Those Leftovers: Use leftover roasted vegetables in frittatas, omelets, blended into soup or as a pizza topping.

 Nice Price: Don't waste money buying fruit and vegetable wash to remove wax, chemicals and soil. Make your own by combining 1 tablespoon of baking soda, one tablespoon of fresh lemon juice and 1 cup of water in a clean spray bottle.

"If I cook, they're gonna have vegetables."

NUTRITION FACTS PER SERVING: 130 calories, 4g total fat, 0.5g saturated fat, 0mg cholesterol, 60mg sodium, 23g carbohydrate, 6g dietary fiber, 7g sugar, 3g protein

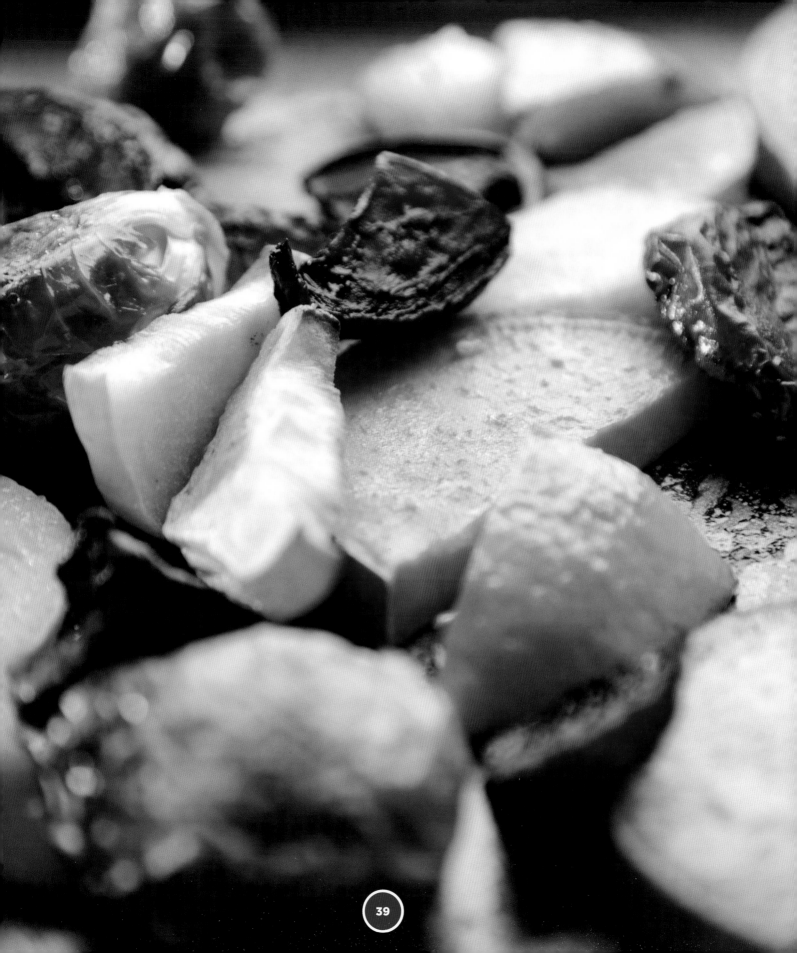

INGREDIENTS:

1 pound Kirby cucumbers, quartered (Kirby cucumbers are usually less than 6-inches long and have bumpy skin and firm flesh. Other cucumbers will work too.)

2 tablespoons kosher or pickling salt (Contains no iodine, added minerals or anticaking agents)

1 tablespoon mustard seeds

2 teaspoons fresh dill weed or 1 teaspoon dill seeds

1 teaspoon coriander seeds

1 teaspoon whole black peppercorns

½ teaspoon red pepper flakes

1 bay leaf

1 garlic clove, peeled and smashed

1 cup white vinegar

½ cup water

2 tablespoons sugar

VARIATIONS:

Quick Pickled Blend: Cut ½ medium head cauliflower into 1-inch florets and 1 red pepper into strips. Prepare recipe the same as cucumber version but substitute cauliflower and red peppers for cucumbers.

Quick Pickled Radishes: Thinly slice 1 pound of radishes. Prepare recipe the same as cucumber version but substitute radishes for cucumbers.

Quick Pickled Okra or Green Beans: Trim the stems of 1 pound of okra or green beans to ½-inch. Prepare recipe the same as cucumber version but substitute okra or green beans for cucumbers, alternate stems up and down.

Quick Pickles

MAKES 8 SERVINGS • SERVING SIZE: 1 SPEAR

Pickling often makes you think of your grandmother, sweating over a steaming pot in late summer as she pickled cucumbers. This quick, easy pickling technique lets you bypass the canning equipment and the hot kitchen. The vinegar and salt add great flavor to these crunchy pickles, which appeal to kids and are cheaper than those sold in stores. Use these individual ingredients to make a homemade pickling spice blend or look for a pre-made spice at the store.

DIRECTIONS:

Thoroughly scrub cucumbers and slice into spears. Pack cucumber spears in a 1-quart glass jar, leaving about ½ inch of space at the top. Set aside.

To make brine (salt water mixture) combine remaining ingredients in a pan over medium heat. Stir until salt and sugar dissolve. Bring to boil.

Pour brine over cucumber spears. Make sure to cover them completely with brine. Let cool 1 hour. Put lid on and shake. Refrigerate 1 day before using. If you can't wait that long, they're still tasty after just a few hours of pickling. Store pickles in the refrigerator and use within one week.

 Kid Friendly: Let kids measure and pour the brine. Even quick pickles require time. This gives kids a chance to learn patience.

 Less Mess: If you make brine in a teapot or pour it into a pitcher, it will be easier to pour into the pickle jars.

 Family Time Around the Table: Share something that makes you 'sour' and something that makes you 'sweet.'

 Love Those Leftovers: Use leftover pickle brine to flavor egg, tuna and potato salads.

 Nice Price: Check the local farmers' market for vegetables you can buy in bulk. Consider going in with others to buy larger quantities. This could be a great time for a pickling party.

"When I buy fruits and vegetables, bring them in and wash them up, my kids will tear them up. It's a lot about what you're bringing home."

NUTRITION FACTS PER SERVING: 4 calories, 0g total fat, 0g saturated fat, 0mg cholesterol, 283mg sodium, 0.84g carbohydrate, 0.4g dietary fiber, 0.37g sugar, 0.18g protein

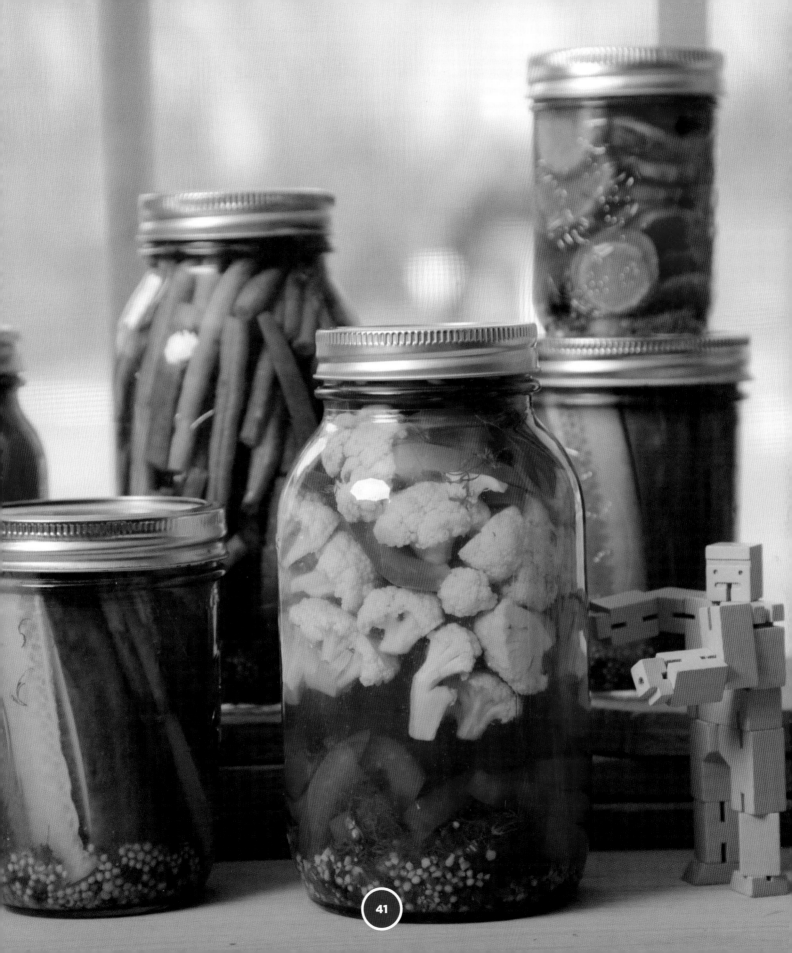

Making Vegetables: Your Way

Here's your chance to join the challenge. Use this cooking guide to help you prepare a whole variety of vegetables for your family. Choose vegetables in season for the tastiest and least expensive results.

VEGETABLE	BOILED	STEAMED	BAKED/ ROASTED	MICROWAVED
Asparagus	Not recommended	8-10 min	400 degrees F for 8-10 min	2-4 min
Beans	6-8 min	5-8 min	425 degrees F for 12-15 min	3-4 min
Brussels Sprouts	Bring to a boil, simmer 5-7 min	8-10 min	400 degrees F for 20 min	4-6 min
Broccoli	4-6 min	5-6 min	425 degrees F for 15-18 min	2-3 min
Cabbage (shredded)	5-10 min	5-8 min	400 degrees F for 30 min (wedges)	5-6 min
Carrots	5-10 min	4-5 min	400 degrees F for 20-30 min (baby carrots)	4-5 min
Cauliflower	5-10 min	5-10 min	400 degrees F for 25-30 min	2-3 min
Corn on the Cob	5-8 min	4-7 min	350 degrees F for 30 min husk on	1.5-2 min
Eggplant	Not recommended	5-6 min	425 degrees F for 25-30 min	2-4 min
Mushrooms	Not recommended	4-5 min	400 degrees F for 25 min	2-3 min
Onions (sliced)	30-50 min (whole, outer layer removed)	5 min	425 degrees F for 25-30 min	Not recommended
Peas	8-12 min	4-5 min	400 degrees F for 20 min	2-3 min
Peppers	Not recommended	2-4 min	450 degrees F for 15 min or until black (peel skin after)	2-3 min
Potatoes (cut)	15-20 min	10-12 min	425 degrees F for 20 min	6-8 min
Spinach	2-5 min	5-6 min	450 degrees F for 3-6 min	1-2 min
Sweet Potato (cubes)	20-30 min	5-7 min	350 degrees F for 20 min	8 min (whole)

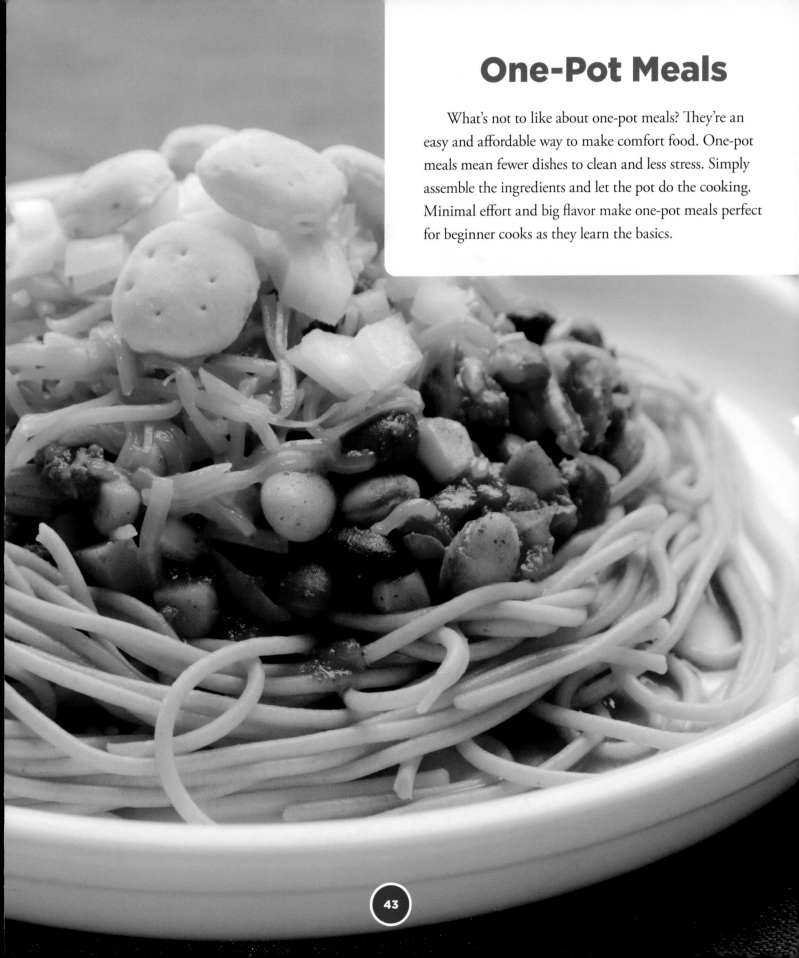

One-Pot Meals

What's not to like about one-pot meals? They're an easy and affordable way to make comfort food. One-pot meals mean fewer dishes to clean and less stress. Simply assemble the ingredients and let the pot do the cooking. Minimal effort and big flavor make one-pot meals perfect for beginner cooks as they learn the basics.

Harvest Chili

MAKES 12 SERVINGS • SERVING SIZE: 1½ CUP

This flavorful chili brings autumn to mind with a mix of vegetables that provide plenty of warm colors. Small cubes of sweet potatoes make a surprise appearance in this one-pot dish. It can easily be made vegetarian, and no one will even notice that the meat is missing. Skipping the meat reduces cost, fat and calories.

INGREDIENTS:

- 1 pound lean ground beef or ground turkey (If you choose not to add meat, you will need 1 tablespoon olive oil to sauté vegetables.)
- 1 medium yellow onion, chopped
- 3 cloves garlic, minced or 1 tablespoon garlic powder (Add the powder with the dried seasonings.)
- 2 green peppers, chopped
- 1 can (28 ounces) diced tomatoes, with liquid (To turn up the heat, use tomatoes with green chilies.)
- 1 medium sweet potato, peeled and chopped
- 3 tablespoons chili powder
  Salt and pepper to your liking
- 1 can (15 ounces) chili beans, with liquid
- 3 cans (15 ounces) tri-bean blend, drained and rinsed (This is a mix of black beans, northern beans, and kidney beans. You can buy one can of each if blend is not available or is more expensive.)
- 1 cup frozen yellow sweet corn, thawed or 1 can (15 ounces) no salt added whole kernel corn, drained and rinsed
- ½ can water, (Use the chili bean can (15 ounces) to capture all the flavoring.)
  Hot sauce, optional

TOPPINGS (optional):

Dollop of plain yogurt, plain Greek yogurt or low-fat sour cream; sliced green onions; shredded cheese; minced jalapeno; chopped cilantro; lime wedges

DIRECTIONS:

In a large pot, cook ground meat, onion, garlic and peppers over medium heat about 10 minutes or until meat is no longer pink. Use a wooden spoon or other utensil to break up large portions of ground meat. Drain.

Add tomatoes, sweet potato and chili powder. Cover and cook until potato is tender, about 15 minutes.

Add beans, corn and water. Reduce heat and simmer uncovered for 30 minutes or until chili reaches desired thickness. Add salt and pepper to your liking. Add hot sauce to kick up the heat.

Add your choice of toppings for additional flavors. Serve.

 Kid Friendly: Allow kids to pick out different toppings for their chili. They will enjoy garnishing their own bowl.

 Less Mess: Bring your recycling bin and trash can close to the kitchen counter so you can toss cans and scraps as you go.

 Family Time Around the Table: Describe how food is grown and what it looks like coming out of the ground.

 Love Those Leftovers: Transform chili into Chili Mac by adding 1 cup of cooked and drained elbow macaroni. For Cincinnati-style chili, add a teaspoon of ground cinnamon when you reheat the chili, then ladle it over cooked and drained spaghetti, top with grated cheddar cheese and onions and serve with crackers.

 Nice Price: Cooking in bulk helps save money. Cook enough chili to feed your family three meals. Eat one meal and freeze the other two. Plan bulk cooking based on what is on sale at the grocery and the coupons you have clipped.

"Cooking makes you feel better about yourself. If you're helping somebody else it makes you feel better. It just kind of gets your mind off of what you've got going on."

NUTRITION FACTS PER SERVING: 200 calories, 2g total fat, 0.5g saturated fat, 25mg cholesterol, 620mg sodium, 18g carbohydrate, 4g dietary fiber, 4g sugar, 13g protein

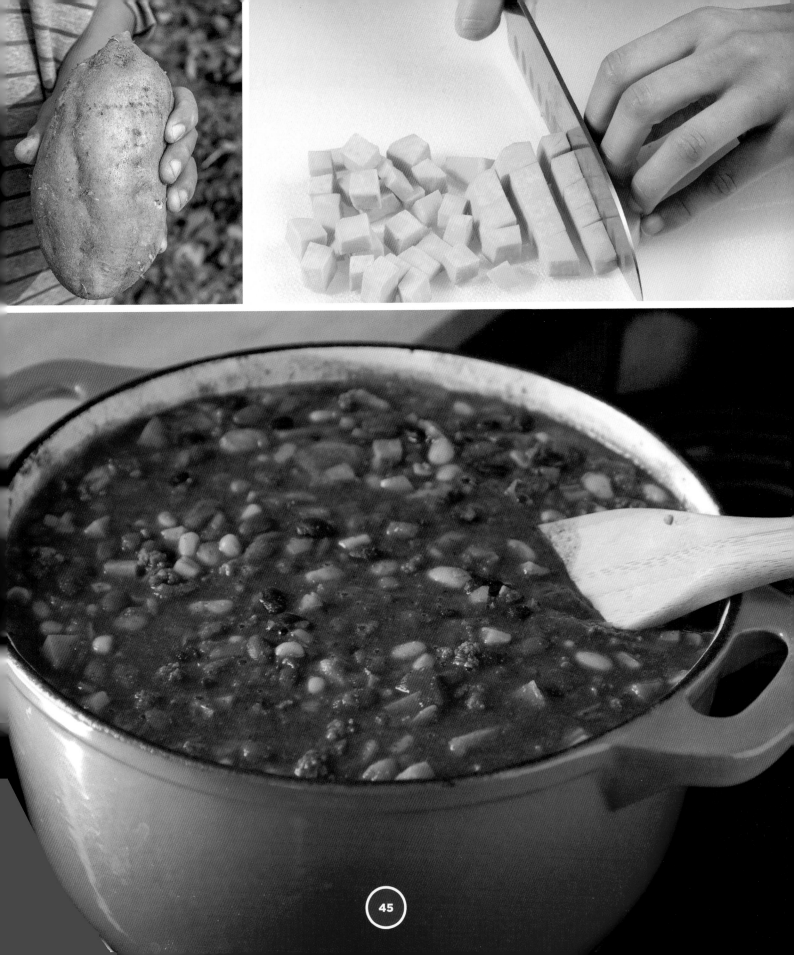

Creamy Broccoli Alfredo

MAKES 6 SERVINGS • SERVING SIZE: 1½ CUP

INGREDIENTS:

- 1 tablespoon butter
- 4 cloves garlic, minced or 4 teaspoons garlic powder (Add garlic powder with the pasta).
- 1½ cups fat-free, low-sodium chicken broth
- 1 cup low-fat milk
- 1 box (8 ounces) fettuccini pasta
- 1 bag (12 ounces) frozen broccoli
- 1 tablespoon cornstarch
- 2 tablespoons cold water
- ⅓ cup grated Parmesan cheese (1 ounce)

Bring a pot of this creamy fettuccine Alfredo to your table and it's sure to become a family favorite. This rich dish can be enjoyed without the guilt because it has less than half the amount of calories and fat of store-bought brands. Most Alfredos are heavy and challenging to make, but not this recipe. It's delicious and easy to prepare.

DIRECTIONS:

In a large pot, sauté garlic in butter over medium-low heat for about 1 minute. Take care not to burn the garlic.

Add chicken broth and milk. Add pasta. Cover and bring to rapid, rolling boil.

Reduce heat to medium low and let pasta simmer, covered, 8-10 minutes or until there is only ½ inch of liquid in bottom of pot. Stir every 2-3 minutes to prevent sticking. Add frozen broccoli and cook, uncovered, until tender.

In a small bowl, combine cornstarch and cold water. Add mixture to pot and return to boil for 1 minute, stirring often.

Remove pot from heat and stir in Parmesan cheese. Serve immediately.

Kid Friendly: Let kids work magic by adding the cornstarch. They can watch as the sauce thickens right before their eyes.

Less Mess: Place the pot in hot soapy water immediately after you serve the pasta. This will soften the cheese and make cleanup much easier.

Family Time Around the Table: Have the kids make a centerpiece for the table and light a candle or turn on battery-powered tea lights. This makes an average night seem like a special occasion.

Love Those Leftovers: Turn the Alfredo into tuna noodle casserole by adding a drained can of tuna. Or reheat with a splash of milk and add cooked chicken, peppers and Cajun spice.

Nice Price: Keep your pantry well stocked with basics such as pasta, tuna and broth. Stock a variety of seasonings. A well-stocked pantry makes it easy to whip up quick, healthy meals and helps you avoid extra trips to the store.

"I want my children to be able to fend for themselves. If something were to ever happen to me I want them to know how to take care of themselves."

NUTRITION FACTS PER SERVING: 210 calories, 4.5g total fat, 2.5g saturated fat, 15mg cholesterol, 220mg sodium, 33g carbohydrate, 4g dietary fiber, 4g sugar, 10g protein

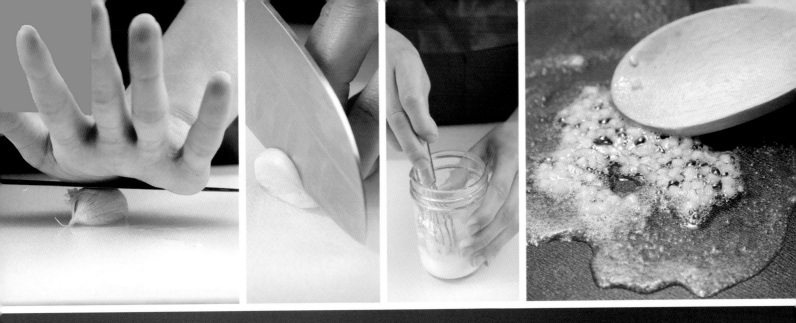

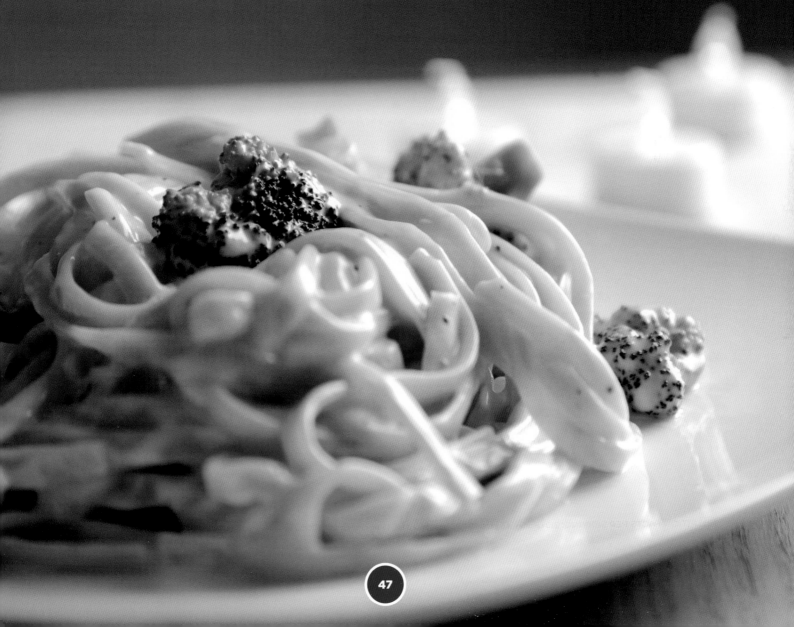

INGREDIENTS:

- 1 tablespoon olive oil
- 1 medium yellow onion, chopped
- 1 pound boneless, skinless chicken breast, chopped into bite-sized pieces
- 1 cup uncooked rice
- 2 cups fat-free, low-sodium chicken broth
- 1 can (14½ ounces) diced tomatoes and chilies
- 1 can (10 ounces) enchilada sauce
- 1 cup frozen yellow sweet corn, thawed or 1 can (15 ounces) no salt added whole kernel corn, drained and rinsed
- 2 teaspoons chili powder
- 1 teaspoon ground cumin
- 1 can (15 ounces) black beans, drained and rinsed

   Salt and pepper to your liking

Southwestern Chicken and Rice

MAKES 8 SERVINGS • SERVING SIZE: 1½ CUP

Enjoy Southwest flavors in this satisfying one-pot chicken and rice dish. Its vivid blend of flavors is tangy but not overly hot. One tester called it "one of those dishes that you crave." Show kids how easy it is to whip up restaurant-style flavor at home. Simple prep and cleanup will leave you less stressed than going out to eat.

DIRECTIONS:

In a large pot, sauté onion in olive oil over medium-high heat about 2 minutes or until tender.

Add chicken and cook 6 minutes or until chicken is no longer pink.

Add rice to pot and stir. Cook 3-4 minutes, stirring occasionally. Chicken and rice should be golden brown.

Add chicken broth, diced tomatoes and chilies, enchilada sauce, corn, chili powder and ground cumin. Stir. Bring liquid to a boil.

Reduce to simmer and cover pot. Cook covered, stirring occasionally. Let cook until rice has absorbed liquid, about 20 minutes. (Brown rice will take longer; about 30 minutes.)

Remove from heat. Add black beans and toss. Serve hot.

Kid Friendly: Show kids the difference between a boil and a simmer. This will remind them how important it is to pay close attention.

Less Mess: Disinfect sponges by rinsing them with soapy water and heating damp sponges in the microwave for 1 minute. Change sponges often.

Family Time Around the Table: Name a famous person you would like to be for a day and why.

Love Those Leftovers: Turn this dish into baked-chicken enchiladas. Spoon mixture into tortillas, roll up and place in baking dish. Pour enchilada sauce over wraps and top with cheese. Bake at 350 degrees F for 15-20 minutes.

Nice Price: Save money by buying one pound of chicken thighs instead of one pound of boneless chicken breasts. Ask the grocery's meat department to debone the chicken thighs. They will usually do this for free.

"I cook at home to feed my kids. I mean the first thing they say when they come home from school is they're hungry."

NUTRITION FACTS PER SERVING: 270 calories, 4.5g total fat, 0.5g saturated fat, 35mg cholesterol, 600mg sodium, 38g carbohydrate, 6g dietary fiber, 6g sugar, 20g protein

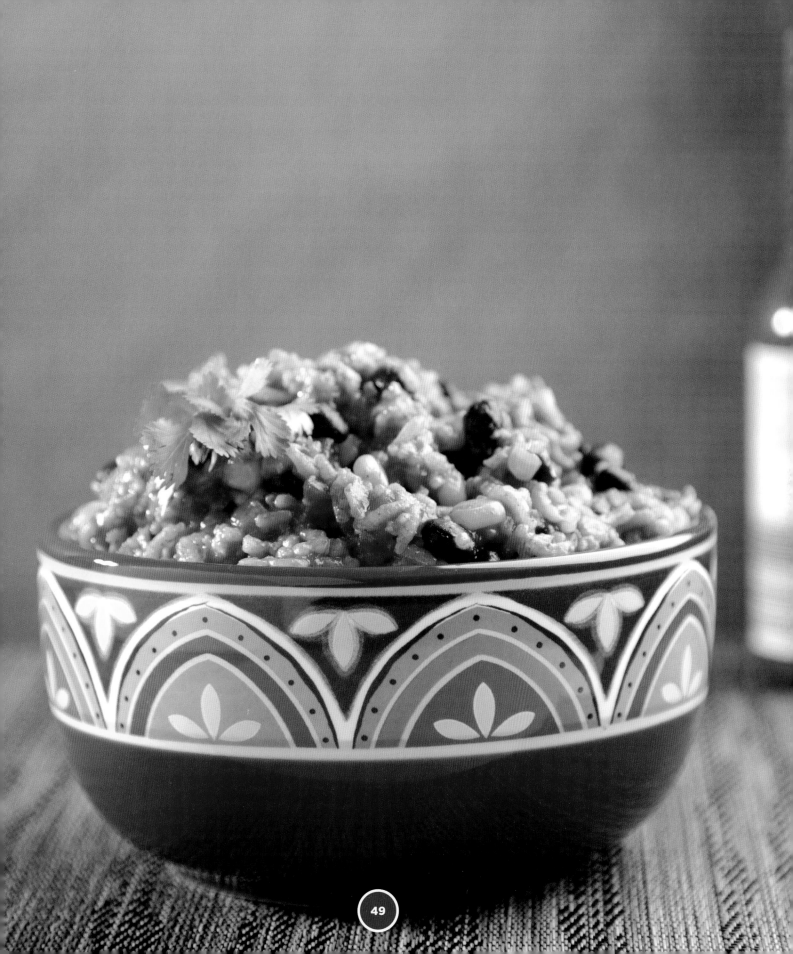

Making One-Pot Meals: More Ways

Now, it's your turn to be creative. Keep in mind that when you prepare your one-pot dish, it is important to include vegetables, whole grains, fat-free or low-fat dairy products and lean protein. Water can be completely or partially replaced by broth or stock to add more flavor. Add vegetables to the pot according to how long it takes them to cook. For example, sturdier vegetables should be added earlier than leaf vegetables. Remember to rinse uncooked pasta or rice in cold water before putting it in the pot. This removes some of the extra starch and keeps the dish from becoming mushy.

After your family sees how easy it is to prepare one-pot meals, you might find you're not the only cook in the kitchen. One pot. One burner. One delicious meal.

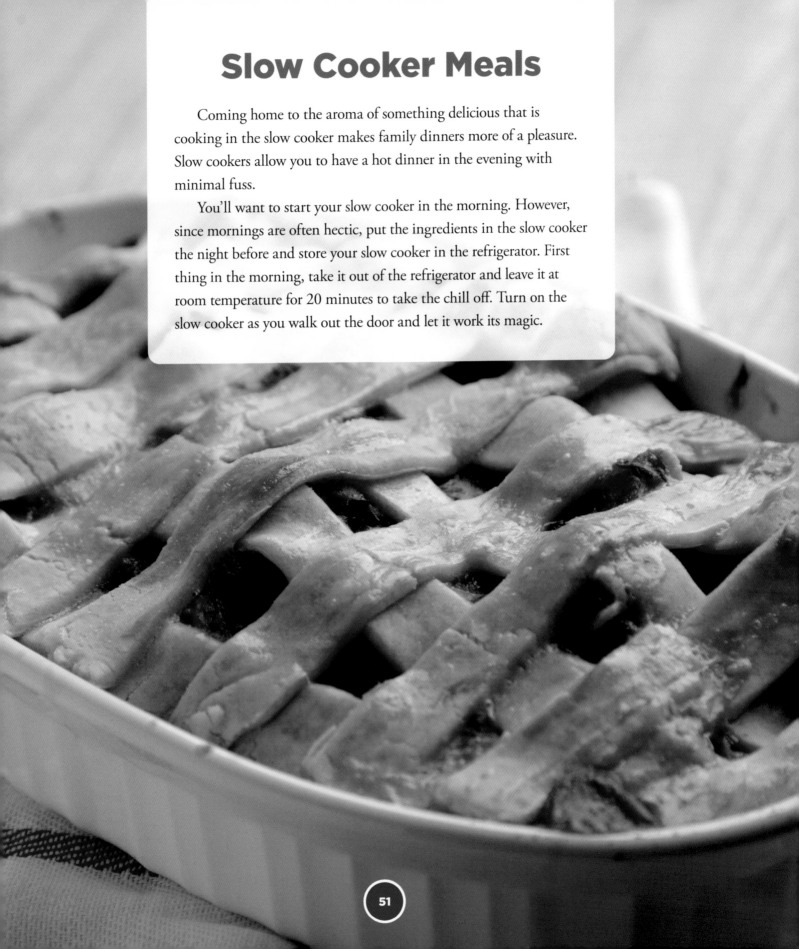

Slow Cooker Meals

Coming home to the aroma of something delicious that is cooking in the slow cooker makes family dinners more of a pleasure. Slow cookers allow you to have a hot dinner in the evening with minimal fuss.

You'll want to start your slow cooker in the morning. However, since mornings are often hectic, put the ingredients in the slow cooker the night before and store your slow cooker in the refrigerator. First thing in the morning, take it out of the refrigerator and leave it at room temperature for 20 minutes to take the chill off. Turn on the slow cooker as you walk out the door and let it work its magic.

Slow Cooker Beef Stew

MAKES 8 SERVINGS • SERVING SIZE: ½ CUP

INGREDIENTS:

- 1½ pounds stew meat
- ½ teaspoon salt
- ½ teaspoon pepper
- 3 tablespoons olive oil
- 1 medium yellow onion, chopped
- 3 cloves garlic, minced or 1 tablespoon garlic powder
- 1 can (4 ounces) tomato paste
- 1 box (32 ounces) low-sodium beef broth
- 6 medium yellow (Yukon) potatoes, chopped, unpeeled
- 4 medium carrots, peeled and chopped
- 1 tablespoon dried thyme leaves
- 1 tablespoon dried rosemary leaves
- 2 bay leaves
- 2 dashes Worcestershire sauce
- 1 tablespoon cornstarch
- 1 tablespoon cold water

Slow cookers make the most of inexpensive cuts of meat, bringing out flavors and softening textures with a long, slow cooking process. They also give the cook some freedom. Turn the slow cooker on and go do whatever you choose.

DIRECTIONS:

Salt and pepper the stew meat.

In a skillet, brown stew meat on all sides, in olive oil, over medium-high heat until the outside has a brown crust, about 2 minutes. Remove meat from skillet; set aside on plate.

Add onions and garlic to skillet, stirring to coat in brown bits from meat. Cook 2 minutes. Add tomato paste. Stir and cook 2 more minutes.

Transfer tomato and onion mixture to a 5-quart slow cooker. Add beef broth, stirring constantly. Add thyme, rosemary, bay leaves and Worcestershire sauce. Add potatoes, carrots and meat.

Cover slow cooker and cook on low 8-10 hours or on high 4-6 hours. At the end of cooking time, combine cornstarch and cold water in a small bowl. Add mixture to the slow cooker and stir for one minute. Serve.

 Kid Friendly: Allow kids to smell and taste the different spices before they are added to the stew. They will become familiar with which spices create which flavors.

 Less Mess: Use baking soda and elbow grease for hard-to-clean, burnt spots on skillets and pans.

 Family Time Around the Table: Put your phones and electronics in another room during mealtime. It can be a relief to have no distractions.

 Love Those Leftovers: Turn your leftover stew into beef potpie. Pour the stew into a pie shell, cover it with a second crust and cut slits into the top. Bake at 350 degrees F for 30 minutes.

 Nice Price: Using a slow cooker allows you to buy cheaper, tougher cuts of meat that will become tender after hours of slow cooking.

"We all find time for each other. And I wouldn't give that up for nothing. I wouldn't give that up for winning the lottery."

NUTRITION FACTS PER SERVING: 240 calories, 9g total fat, 2.5g saturated fat, 55mg cholesterol, 430mg sodium, 18g carbohydrate, 3g dietary fiber, 5g sugar, 22g protein

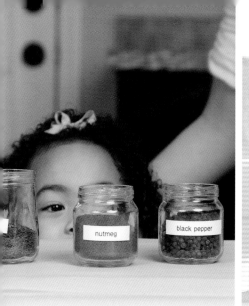

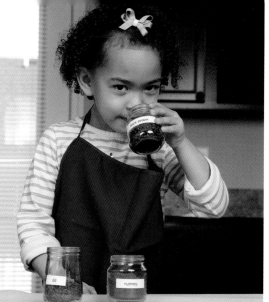

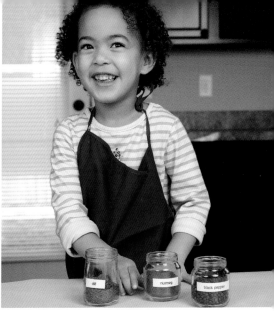

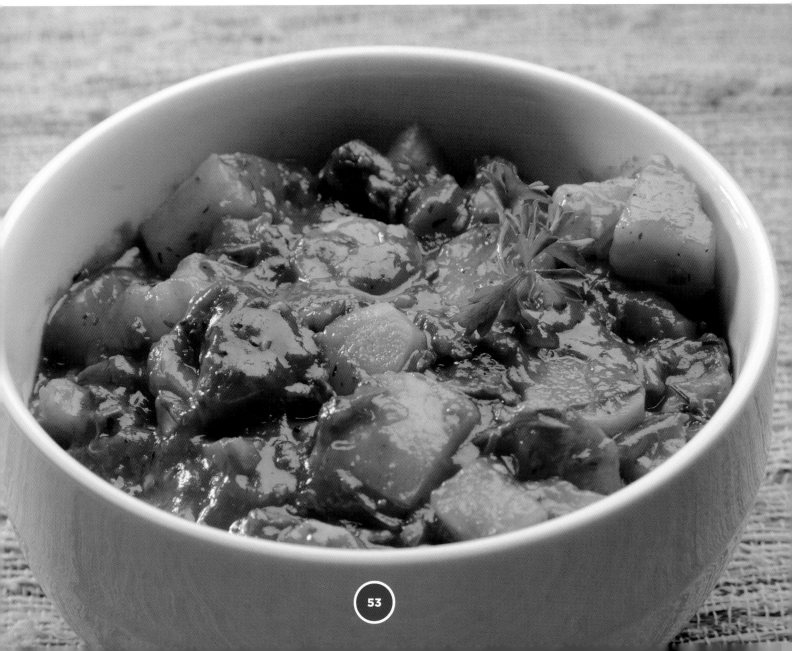

Slow Cooker Barbecue Chicken

MAKES 10 SERVINGS • SERVING SIZE: ½ CUP PULLED CHICKEN

Chicken thighs are inexpensive and have great flavor. Add barbecue sauce and a long, slow cooking process, and you've got a recipe for something special.

INGREDIENTS:

- 8 bone-in chicken thighs (about 3 pounds)
- Salt and pepper
- 3 cloves garlic, minced or 1 tablespoon garlic powder
- 2 teaspoons prepared yellow mustard
- ½ cup honey or brown sugar
- ⅛-½ teaspoon hot sauce
- 2 teaspoons Worcestershire sauce
- 1 tablespoon cornstarch

DIRECTIONS:

Salt and pepper chicken.

Place chicken on a broiling pan or cooling rack atop a cookie sheet. Place pan in oven on middle rack and broil chicken thighs 3-4 minutes per side or until lightly browned. Transfer to 5-quart slow cooker.

In a small bowl, combine remaining ingredients and spoon over chicken to coat.

In the slow cooker, cover and cook on low 8 hours or on high 4-6 hours. Chicken will be tender and should fall off the bone.

 Kid Friendly: Help kids shred the chicken after it has cooked and cooled. This teaches them how you can change the texture of food.

 Less Mess: Use slow cooker liners to save time and energy.

 Family Time Around the Table: Name three things you can't live without and why.

 Love Those Leftovers: Use leftover barbecue chicken as a pizza topping.

 Nice Price: Watch for deals on chicken thighs and freeze extras. Remove packaging, rewrap food in plastic wrap and place in a freezer bag. Mark the bag with the date the chicken was frozen.

"I want to cook healthy food but I still want it to have that 'pow!' effect, like you get in soul food cooking."

NUTRITION FACTS PER SERVING: 180 calories, 6g total fat, 2g saturated fat, 105mg cholesterol, 105mg sodium, 11g carbohydrate, 0g dietary fiber, 8g sugar, 19g protein

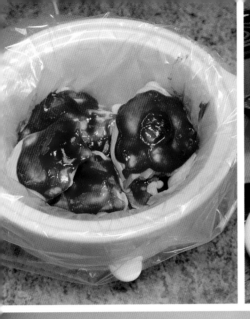
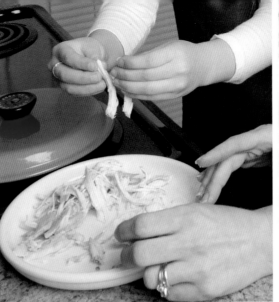
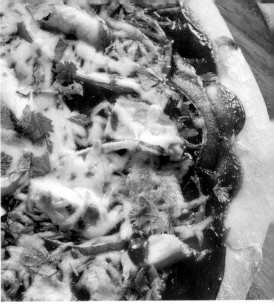
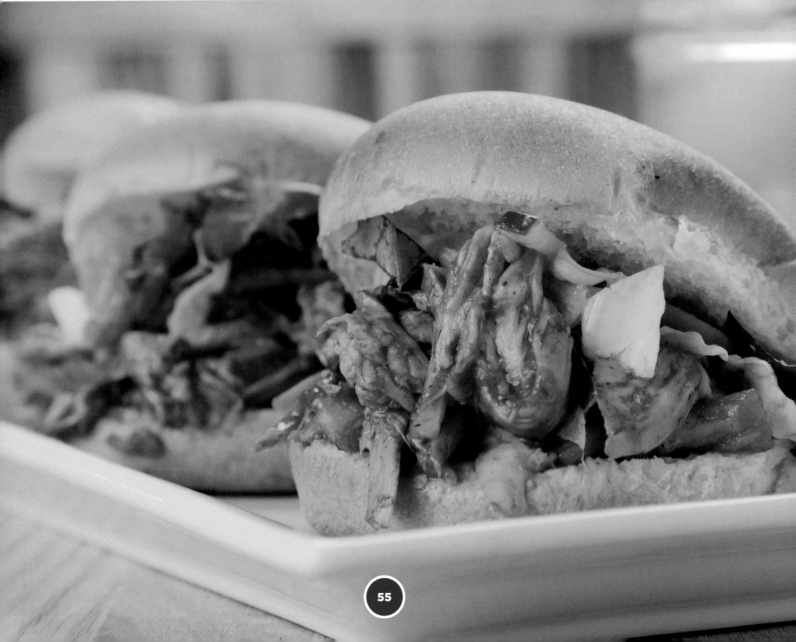

INGREDIENTS:

- 2 tablespoons olive oil
- 3 cloves garlic, minced or 1 tablespoon garlic powder
- 1 medium yellow onion, chopped
- 4 stalks celery, chopped
- 1 pound dried pinto or white beans, sorted and rinsed
- 1 teaspoon dried thyme leaves
- 1 teaspoon dried rosemary leaves
- 2 bay leaves
- ½ teaspoon ground paprika
- 6 cups water

  Salt and pepper to your liking

TOPPINGS (optional):

Shredded cheese, chopped onions, chopped tomatoes, crumbled cornbread, chow-chow and/or pickle relish

Slow Cooker Soup Beans

MAKES 8 SERVINGS • SERVING SIZE: 1½ CUPS

Soup beans are easy and extra delicious when they are prepared in a slow cooker. And beans are one of the most affordable, filling sources of protein around. Serve this dish with cornbread and greens and you'll have what Kentuckians call "good eating."

DIRECTIONS:

In a 5-quart slow cooker, add olive oil, garlic, onion and celery.

Sort through beans and remove debris or stones. Rinse beans; add beans and remaining seasonings to slow cooker.

Add water, stir and combine ingredients. Cover and cook on low 8 hours or on high 4 hours.

Mash beans slightly. Add salt and pepper to your liking.

Add your choice of toppings for additional flavor. Serve.

 Kid Friendly: Let kids sort and rinse the beans before putting them in the slow cooker. They will learn how to find rocks or rotten beans that must be removed.

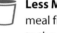 **Less Mess:** After you remove your meal from the slow cooker, add water to the slow cooker and turn it on low to make cleanup easier.

 Family Time Around the Table: Share a favorite poem or song lyrics.

 Love Those Leftovers: Turn soup beans into refried beans. Mash some of the beans with a potato masher and add them to a hot, oiled skillet. Add chili and garlic powder to your liking. Cook until heated.

 Nice Price: Have beans for dinner at least once a week to give your food budget a boost.

"My daughter loves to do things for people. She'll make simple, homemade dishes and bring a plate to our neighbors."

NUTRITION FACTS PER SERVING: 240 calories, 3.5g total fat, 0.5g saturated fat, 0mg cholesterol, 30mg sodium, 39g carbohydrate, 14g dietary fiber, 4g sugar, 12grams protein

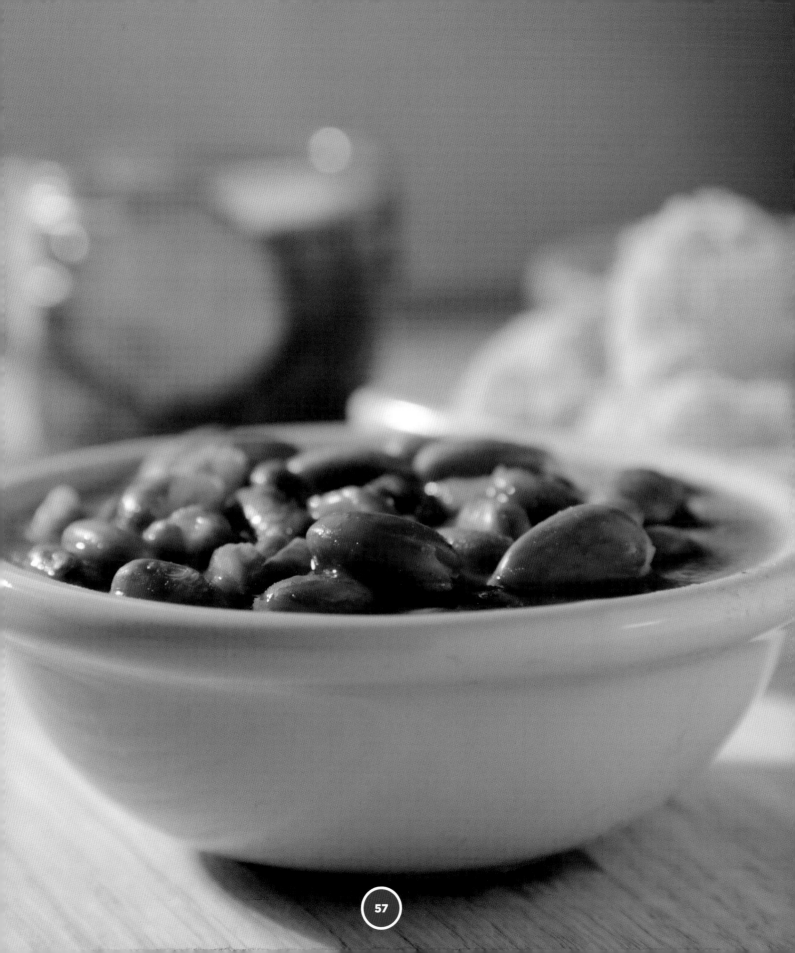

Slow Cooker Meals: Your Way

Your slow cooker may soon become your favorite appliance. It offers you and your family the comfort of healthy, home cooked meals even on busy weekdays. The minimal mess and little supervision make this a favorite kitchen companion.

Here are a few more tips to help make using your slow cooker even easier.

Slow Cooker Tips

◆ Choose the right size slow cooker for your family and prepare recipes accordingly:

> Small: 1½, 2 and 2½ quart capacity

> Medium: 3, 3½, 4 and 4½ quart capacity

> Large: 5, 5½, 6 and 7 quart capacity.

◆ Brown meat and/or vegetables before placing them in the slow cooker to add extra flavor.

◆ Thaw frozen meat, poultry and other ingredients in the refrigerator before adding them to the slow cooker.

◆ When you place meat in the slow cooker, leave space between pieces of meat so the heat can circulate around them.

◆ Do not overfill the slow cooker. Fill to at least half full but no more than two-thirds full.

◆ Cut meat into smaller pieces so the pieces will cook throughout.

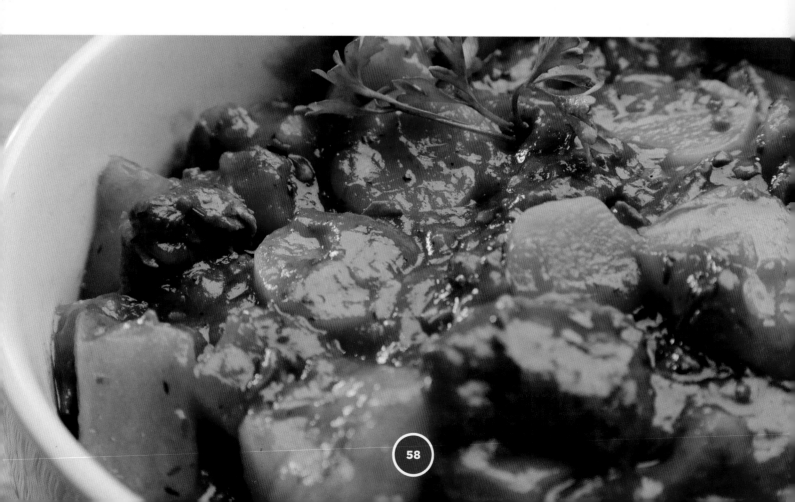

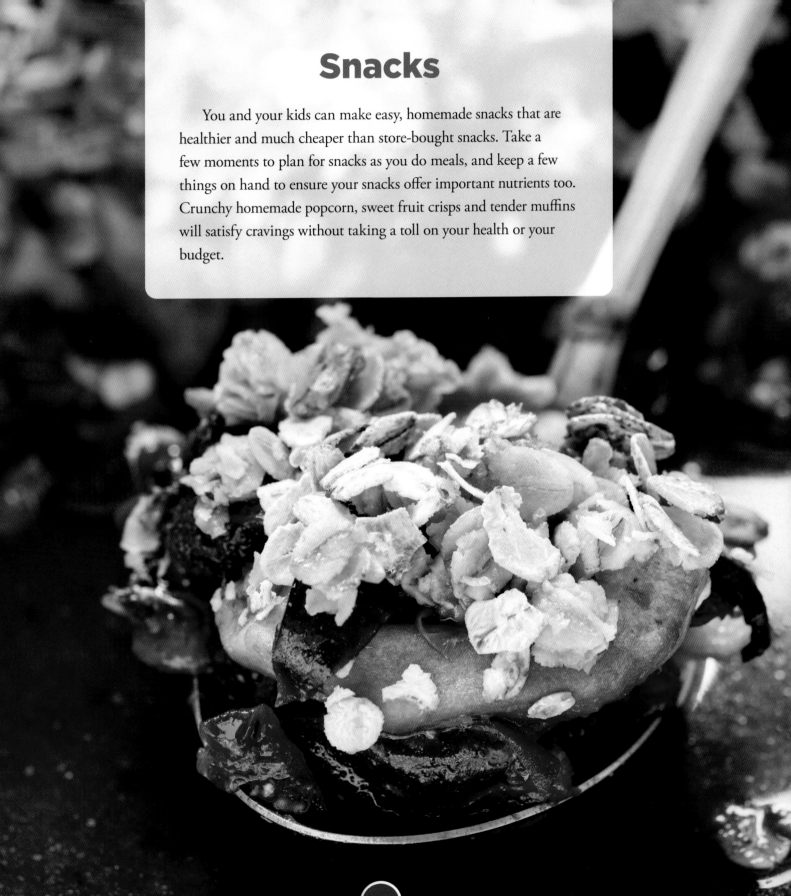

Snacks

You and your kids can make easy, homemade snacks that are healthier and much cheaper than store-bought snacks. Take a few moments to plan for snacks as you do meals, and keep a few things on hand to ensure your snacks offer important nutrients too. Crunchy homemade popcorn, sweet fruit crisps and tender muffins will satisfy cravings without taking a toll on your health or your budget.

Stovetop Popcorn

MAKES 8 SERVINGS • SERVING SIZE: 2 CUP

You can make popcorn in a pan almost as fast as you can make expensive microwave popcorn. Kids love making popcorn on the stove because it seems like magic as the hard corn kernels turn into fluffy popcorn. Stovetop popcorn is a fluffy, crunchy, whole-grain snack that makes any ordinary night more fun. Try the variations we offer here or create your own.

INGREDIENTS:

- 2 tablespoons vegetable oil
- ½ cup popcorn kernels
- 2 tablespoons butter, melted
- Salt to your liking

VARIATIONS:

Cool Ranch Popcorn: Add 2 tablespoons powdered buttermilk, 2 tablespoons ground black pepper and 2 teaspoons dried dill weed.

Chili Popcorn: Add 2 tablespoons chili powder.

Cinnamon Sugar Popcorn: Mix together ¼ cup sugar and ¼ cup ground cinnamon and add to popcorn.

DIRECTIONS:

In a large pot, heat vegetable oil and 3 kernels of popcorn over medium-high heat. Cover with a tight-fitting lid. As soon as kernels pop, add remaining kernels in an even layer. Cover again.

Use pot holders to shake pot from side-to-side over the burner. The moment popcorn starts to pop, turn the heat down to medium-low and continue to gently shake.

After popping slows to 3-5 seconds between pops, remove pot from heat, remove lid and put popcorn into a wide bowl. Add melted butter and salt to popcorn. Toss gently.

MICROWAVE METHOD:

The easiest and least expensive way to pop corn is to put ¼ cup plain popcorn in a lunch size brown paper bag. Fold the top of the bag twice and place it fold side down in the microwave. No oil needed. Cook on high for 2 minutes or until the popping sound stops. Add spray butter and seasonings if you like.

 Kid Friendly: Kids will have fun listening for the popping sound. They will learn that cooking involves all the senses, including hearing.

 Less Mess: Pour popcorn into a bowl before adding butter or seasoning so nothing sticks to the hot pan. Toss popcorn with clean hands or salad tongs.

 Family Time Around the Table: Describe one way you helped another person today.

 Love Those Leftovers: Add leftover popcorn to trail mix or make popcorn balls. Melt 2 tablespoons of peanut butter in a microwave or on the stove. Add ½ cup of dried fruit, and fold in 2 cups of popcorn. Cool slightly. Form mixture into balls and let sit for 2-4 hours.

 Nice Price: Don't waste money on prebagged or microwaved popcorn. This recipe costs about $1 to make and feeds four.

"And this is what my mother always told me, when cooking… you gotta listen."

NUTRITION FACTS PER SERVING: 100 calories, 7g total fat, 2g saturated fat, 10mg cholesterol, 25mg sodium, 10g carbohydrate, 1g dietary fiber, 0g sugar, 1g protein

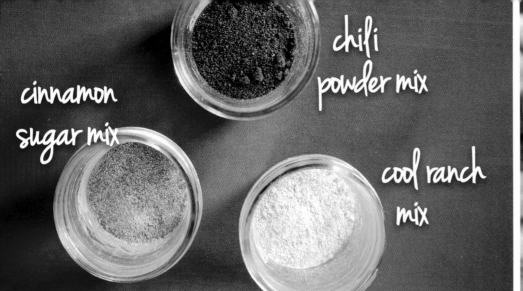

cinnamon
sugar mix

chili
powder mix

cool ranch
mix

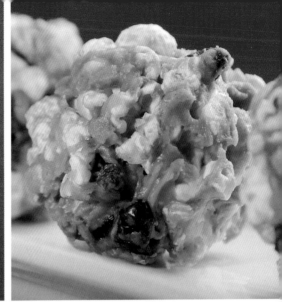

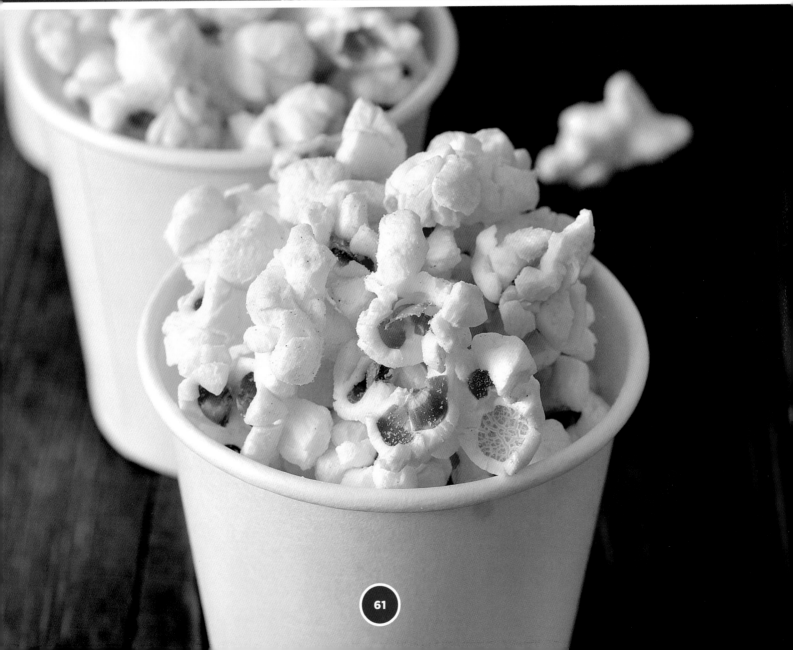

61

INGREDIENTS:

Nonstick spray

3   medium apples, peeled and sliced

2   tablespoons sugar

1   teaspoon cornstarch

1½ teaspoons water

½   teaspoon lemon juice

½   cup old-fashioned oats

¼   cup all-purpose flour

¼   cup brown sugar, packed

½   teaspoon ground cinnamon

¼   cup cold butter

VARIATIONS:

Blueberry and Apricot Crisp: Cut up 6 apricots and combine with ½ pint blueberries. Prepare recipe the same as apple version but substitute blueberries and apricots for apples.

Peach Crisp: Cut up 4 peaches. Prepare recipe the same as apple version but substitute peaches for apples.

Mixed Berry Crisp: Prepare recipe the same as apple version but substitute 3 cups mixed berries for apples.

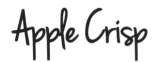

Apple Crisp

MAKES 8 SERVINGS • SERVING SIZE: ⅛ OF CRISP

Sweet and crunchy fruit crisps are a simple way to serve a homemade, baked treat anytime. This warm apple crisp is a family favorite, with its gooey insides and crumbly topping. Feel free to use seasonal fruits or any fruit you have on hand—fresh, frozen or canned.

DIRECTIONS:

Preheat oven to 375 degrees F.

Prepare 1-quart baking dish with nonstick spray. Place sliced apples in baking dish.

In a small bowl, combine sugar, cornstarch, water and lemon juice until smooth. Pour over apples.

Combine oats, flour, brown sugar and ground cinnamon; cut in butter until mixture is crumbly. Sprinkle over apples.

Bake 20-25 minutes or until filling is bubbly. Let cool and serve.

 Kid Friendly: Teach kids how to cut the butter into the flour and oat mixture. This is an important baking skill.

 Less Mess: After you finish the apples, use the same bowl to mix the crumble.

 Family Time Around the Table: Describe yourself in three positive words.

 Love Those Leftovers: Use leftover crisp to top oatmeal.

 Nice Price: This recipe can be made from most fruits. Buy a cheaper type of fruit if those mentioned above are too pricey.

*"My grandmother never measures anything.
She is a smell, taste, see type of cook."*

NUTRITION FACTS PER SERVING: 160 calories, 6g total fat, 3.5g saturated fat, 15mg cholesterol, 0mg sodium, 24g carbohydrate, 2g dietary fiber, 16g sugar, 2g protein

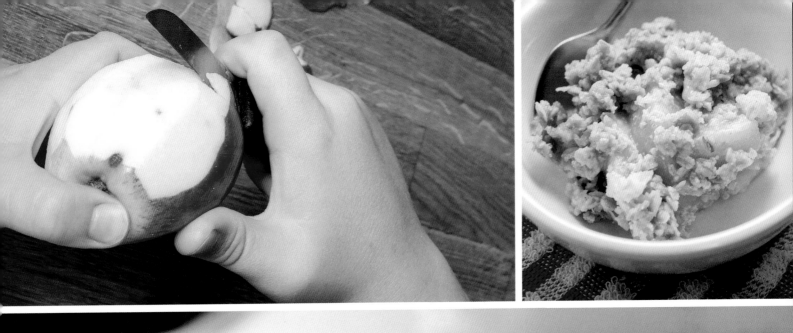

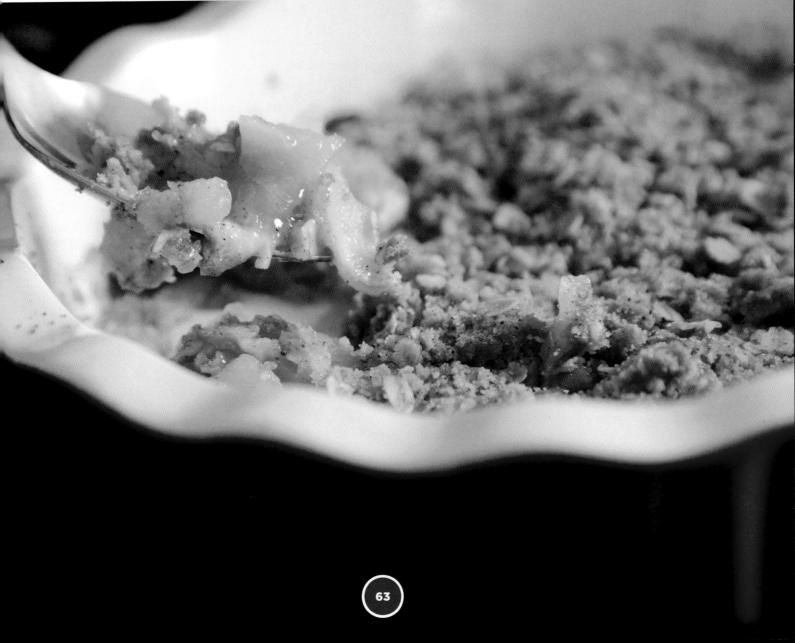

INGREDIENTS:

Nonstick spray

2	cups all-purpose flour, sifted
1	tablespoon baking powder
½	teaspoon salt
5	tablespoons sugar
1	egg
1	cup low-fat milk
4	tablespoons butter, melted

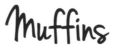

Muffins

MAKES 12 SERVINGS • SERVING SIZE: 1 MUFFIN

Even if the pantry is almost bare, chances are good you still have the staples needed to make warm, homemade muffins. By using fruits and other ingredients you have on hand, you can make an endless variety of muffins. Let kids choose the add-ins and name their creations: Jacob's Jammin' Muffins, Keisha's Awesomesauce Mini Muffins, and Mom's NeedsaBreak-FAST Muffins.

VARIATIONS:

Blueberry Orange Muffins: Add 1 cup fresh or frozen blueberries, zest of one orange and juice of half of the orange when stirring the egg mixture into the dry ingredients. To zest, use a vegetable peeler and paring knife, or a box grater to take off the outermost layer of the fruit's peel.

Oatmeal Applesauce Muffins: Add 1 ½ cups rolled oats, 1 teaspoon baking soda, 1 teaspoon ground cinnamon and ½ cup brown sugar to dry ingredients. Add 1 cup applesauce and 3 tablespoons oil to the egg mixture.

Lemon Poppy Seed Muffins: Instead of 5 tablespoons sugar, add 1 cup sugar to dry ingredients. Add ¼ cup poppy seeds, ⅓ cup corn oil, ¼ cup lemon juice and an additional egg (total of 2 eggs) to the egg mixture.

DIRECTIONS:

Preheat oven to 400 degrees F.

Prepare muffin tins with nonstick spray.

In a large bowl, sift together flour, baking powder, salt and sugar. In another bowl, beat together egg, milk and melted butter.

Pour flour mixture into egg mixture. Stir quickly and just enough to moisten dry ingredients. Do not over mix.

Fill prepared muffin tins ¾ full with batter. Bake 22 minutes or until muffins are golden brown.

 Kid Friendly: Teach kids to sift. Let them put the flour through the sifter or use a whisk or a fork to add air to flour. This reminds them of the importance of loosening ingredients that have been sitting for too long.

 Less Mess: Use cupcake liners so muffins come out easily and to keep the muffin tins clean.

 Family Time Around the Table: Ask each person to tell a joke.

 Love Those Leftovers: Use leftover muffins to make bread pudding. Combine 2 cups of sugar, 5 eggs, 2 cups of milk, and 2 teaspoons of vanilla extract and pour over 3 cups of cubed muffins. (Stale bread will also work.) Let stand for 10 minutes or as long as 2 hours. Pour mixture into a greased pan and bake for 35 minutes at 350 degrees F.

 Nice Price: Butter freezes well. Take advantage of a sale and buy an extra box to freeze.

"We use cooking as a major educational tool for learning measurements and following directions at our house."

NUTRITION FACTS PER SERVING: 140 calories, 4g total fat, 2.5g saturated fat, 25mg cholesterol, 250mg sodium, 20g carbohydrate, 1g dietary fiber, 5g sugar, 4g protein

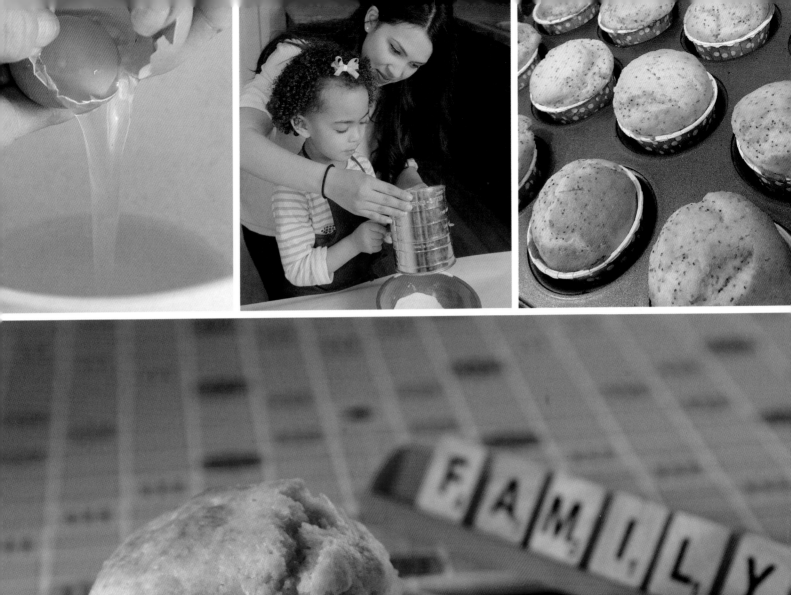
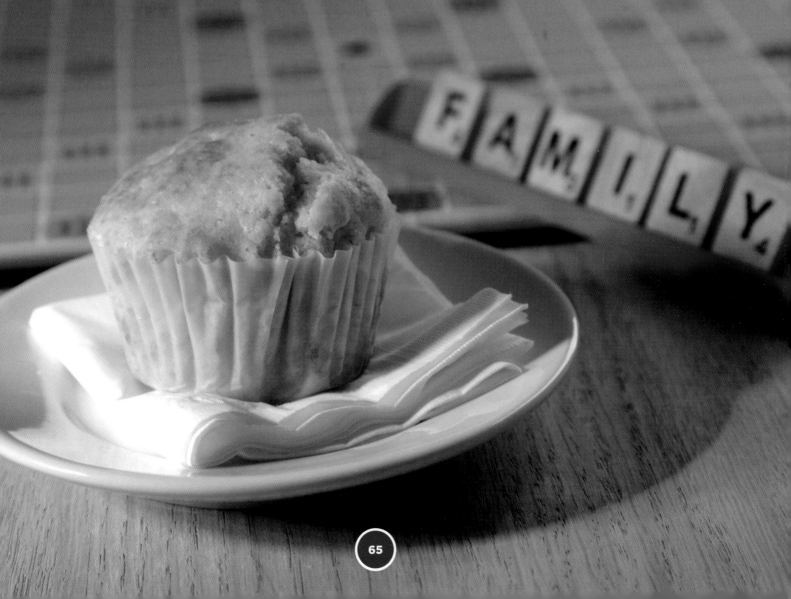

Grab & Go Snacks

Whether eaten on the go or at home, healthy snacks can be easy and quick. You can use pantry staples to make nourishing and delicious bites that ward off hunger between meals. Making snacks at home also teaches kids to be resourceful and creative.

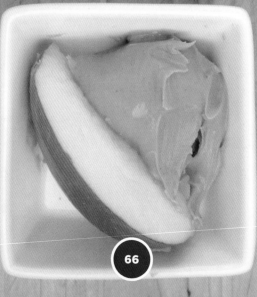

power up – sunflower seeds and raisins

cheese and crackers

fruit kebobs

peanut butter and apples

Kentucky Proud Produce Availability

Buying Kentucky Proud is easy. Look for the label at your grocery store, farmers' market, or roadside stand. Our secret ingredient is the hard work and dedication of Kentucky's farm families. Find out why "Nothing else is close."

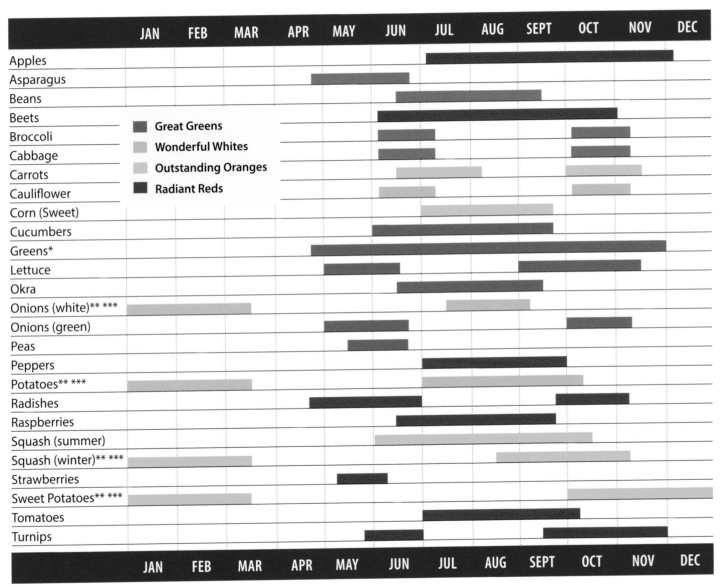

	JAN	FEB	MAR	APR	MAY	JUN	JUL	AUG	SEPT	OCT	NOV	DEC
Apples							■	■	■	■	■	
Asparagus				■	■	■						
Beans						■	■	■	■			
Beets						■	■	■	■	■		
Broccoli						■	■			■	■	
Cabbage						■	■			■	■	
Carrots						■	■	■		■	■	
Cauliflower						■	■			■		
Corn (Sweet)							■	■	■			
Cucumbers						■	■	■	■			
Greens*				■	■	■	■	■	■	■	■	
Lettuce					■	■						
Okra						■	■	■	■			
Onions (white)** ***	■	■	■					■	■			
Onions (green)					■	■				■	■	
Peas					■	■						
Peppers							■	■	■	■		
Potatoes** ***	■	■	■				■	■	■	■		
Radishes				■	■	■				■	■	
Raspberries							■	■	■			
Squash (summer)						■	■	■	■			
Squash (winter)** ***	■	■	■					■	■	■	■	
Strawberries					■							
Sweet Potatoes** ***	■	■	■							■	■	■
Tomatoes							■	■	■	■		
Turnips						■	■		■	■	■	

Legend:
- Great Greens
- Wonderful Whites
- Outstanding Oranges
- Radiant Reds

* Greens refer to any number of different plants including the traditional spinach, mustard, collard, turnip, etc., as well as newer Asian varieties and Swiss chard. ** Storage crops. *** Through the use of season extension methods many of the availability dates are commonly extended in either direction for many of these crops.

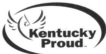
Kentucky Proud.

Youth Friendly Kitchen Tasks

AGE LEVEL	TASK(S)
All Ages	• wash hands
Toddlers:	• help choose fruits and vegetables when shopping • help wash fruits and vegetables with supervision • pick herb leaves off stems • stir • put trash in wastebasket
Preschoolers (in addition to above):	• put small, unbreakable items in the grocery cart or basket • tear lettuce • squeeze a lemon or lime • pour liquids from a small container into glasses • whisk • cut soft ingredients with a plastic knife • wipe up spills • help set and clear table
Elementary school students (in addition to above):	• help plan a meal • find coupons for shopping and match them with products at the store • help find items on grocery and farmers' market lists • use simple equipment with adult supervision (i.e. microwave, blender, etc.) • use measuring spoons and cups • use a grater • break eggs • read recipes out loud • help dry dishes • help unload dishwasher • help prepare school lunch • wipe tables, chairs, counters and stove top • sweep the floor • empty small wastebaskets into trash bag
Middle school students (in addition to above):	• help find the best price when shopping • help put away groceries • check expiration dates and throw out old food • safely use a chef's knife with supervision • use can opener and pizza cutter • pour drinks for meals • put away leftovers • help hand-wash dishes • help load and start dishwasher • clean and disinfect the sink • wipe down inside of microwave • mop the floor • take out trash and recycling

Guide to Portion Sizes

One serving of fruits or vegetables is equal to:

- 1 cup of raw leafy vegetables (10 calories)
- ½ cup of cooked vegetables (20 calories)
- ¾ cup of fruit or vegetable juice (90 calories)
- 1 medium apple, banana, orange, or pear (90 calories)
- ¼ cup dried fruit (109 calories)

One ounce equivalent of grains is equal to:

- 1 slice of bread (70 calories)
- About 1 cup of ready-to-eat cereal (plain corn flakes = 100 calories)
- ½ cup cooked cereal, rice, or pasta (95 calories)
- ½ hotdog or hamburger bun (62 calories)

A serving of meat or beans is equal to:

- 2 to 3 ounces of cooked meat, poultry, or fish (3 ounces lean beef = 143 calories)
- ¼ cup of cooked dry beans = 1 ounce meat (105 calories)
- ⅓ cup of nuts = 1 ounce meat (260 calories)
- 1 egg = 1 ounce meat (80 calories)

One serving of milk is equal to:

- 1 cup of milk or yogurt (1 cup skim milk = 90 calories)
- 1½ ounces of cheese (155 calories)

Measurements and Substitutions

MEASUREMENTS				
3 teaspoons	=	1 tablespoon		
4 tablespoons	=	¼ cup	=	2 fluid ounces
5⅓ tablespoons	=	⅓ cup		
8 tablespoons	=	½ cup	=	4 fluid ounces
16 tablespoons	=	1 cup	=	8 fluid ounces
4 cups	=	1 quart	=	32 fluid ounces

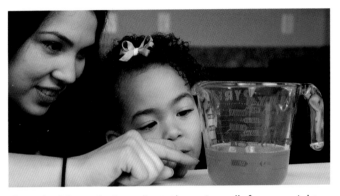

If you don't have the ingredients the recipe calls for, you might be able to use one of the substitutions listed here:

SUBSTITUTIONS	
If you don't have...	**Use...**
1 cup self-rising flour	1 cup all-purpose flour plus 1½ teaspoons baking powder and ½ teaspoon salt
1 cup cake flour	1 cup sifted all-purpose flour minus 2 tablespoons
1 cup all-purpose flour	1 cup cake flour plus 2 tablespoons
1 teaspoon baking powder	½ teaspoon cream of tartar plus ¼ teaspoon baking soda
1 tablespoon cornstarch	2 tablespoons all-purpose flour
2 large eggs	3 small eggs
1 cup yogurt	1 cup buttermilk or 1 cup sour cream
1 cup buttermilk or sour milk	1 tablespoon vinegar or lemon juice plus milk to equal 1 cup

Knife Skills

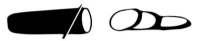

How to Hold a Knife

Basic culinary skills are not learned through osmosis but through practice. It's important to spend a little time on the basics so you can keep improving. Let's get an edge on knife safety and learn how to make your food presentation look sharp.

It is essential to use the right knife to produce the desired cut. The knife should be held firmly in your hand. Always cut away from your body. A wood or polyethylene cutting board improves knife control and reduces the wear on your knife blade. A sharp knife requires less pressure, decreasing the likelihood of slippage and a tired hand.

Top View	Side View
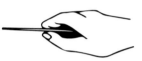	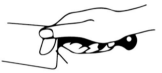

Note the position of finger behind the blade for support.

The correct way to hold a French or chef's knife requires you to hold the knife handle behind the blade while curling your fingers in and around the handle. It's perfect for chopping, slicing, and dicing because the blade is wide at the heel and tapers to a point. The knife actually acts as your guide. Keeping the tip of your knife on the cutting board and slicing down with a rocking motion gives you more control and reduces the risk of cuts.

Illustrations from Cooking a World of New Tastes, Segment 1
http://www.fns.usda.gov/tn/Resources/worldtastes02Seg1.pdf

How to Slice and Dice

Slice Crosswise
Cut vegetable crosswise to the desired thickness

Slice Lengthwise
Cut vegetable lengthwise to the desired thickness

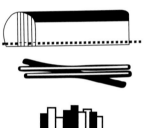

Julienne
Stack slices and cut again lengthwise to the desired thickness

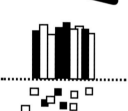

Dice
Lay julienne in a bundle and cut crosswise to the desired thickness

Illustrations from Cooking a World of New Tastes, Segment 1
http://www.fns.usda.gov/tn/Resources/worldtastes02Seg1.pdf

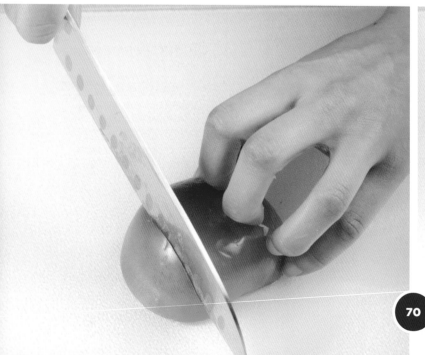

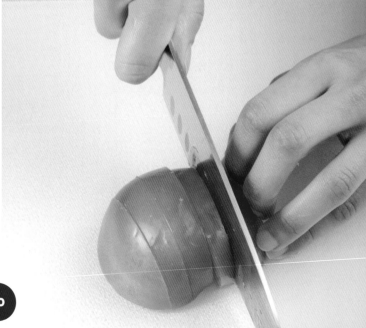

Herbs and Spices: Your Way

Use this handy list of herbs and spices to add flavor like a pro.

SPICE/HERB	FLAVOR	PRODUCE	PROTEINS	USE IN	PAIRS WELL WITH
Bay leaves	bitter, woodsy	mushrooms, potatoes, tomatoes	beans, beef, chicken, lentils, shellfish	foods that require slow cooking, soups, stews marinades, sauces	oregano, parsley, thyme, tarragon
Cayenne pepper	spicy, warm	bell peppers, corn, eggplant, potatoes, tomatoes, zucchini	chicken, beans, beef, eggs, fish	marinades, rice, salad dressings, sauces, soups, stews	cinnamon, cumin, paprika
Cumin	earthy, smoky	carrots, corn, eggplant, green beans, tomatoes, zucchini	beans, beef, cheese, chicken, fish, lentils, pork, tofu	breads, curries, dry rubs, marinades, rice, sauces, soups	basil, cayenne pepper, celery seed, cilantro, cinnamon, dill weed, garlic powder, ginger, oregano, paprika
Garlic powder	strong flavor, warm	Brussels sprouts, cabbage, mushrooms, potatoes, spinach, squash, tomatoes, zucchini	beans, beef, cheese, chicken, fish, tofu	breads, marinades, salad dressings, sauces, stir-fries, soups, stews	basil, celery seed, cilantro, coriander, cumin, dill weed, ginger, lemon, mustard seeds, oregano, paprika, parsley, rosemary, tarragon, thyme
Ginger	sweet, warm	carrots, citrus fruits, sweet potatoes, squash	beef, chicken, fish, pork, tofu	marinades, rice, stir-fries, salad dressings	celery seed, cinnamon, cumin, dill weed, garlic powder, nutmeg
Rosemary	earthy, piney	carrots, mushrooms, parsnips, potatoes, sweet potatoes, tomatoes, turnips	beans, beef, cheese, chicken, fish, pork	breads, marinades, salad dressings, sauces, soups, stews	basil, celery seed, garlic powder, lemon, oregano, parsley, thyme
Thyme	earthy, woodsy	carrots, cauliflower, green beans, mushrooms, parsnips, potatoes, sweet potatoes, tomatoes, turnips	beans, beef, cheese, chicken, fish, lentils, pork	breads, marinades, salad dressings, sauces, soup	basil, bay leaves, celery seed, garlic powder, lemon, nutmeg, oregano, parsley, rosemary, tarragon
Basil	sweet	bell pepper, eggplant, potatoes, tomatoes, zucchini	cheese, chicken, fish, pork	marinades, salad dressings, sauces, soups	chili powder, cinnamon, cumin, dill weed, garlic powder, lemon, oregano, parsley, rosemary, tarragon, thyme
Cinnamon	sweet	apples, carrots, sweet potatoes, squash	chicken	batters, breads, desserts, oatmeal	basil, cayenne pepper, ginger, nutmeg, paprika
Nutmeg	sweet	asparagus, broccoli, cabbage, carrots, cranberries, parsnips, peaches, pumpkin, sweet potatoes, squash, turnips, yams	beans	breads, rice, sauces	cinnamon, coriander seeds, ginger, thyme
Oregano	earthy	artichokes, bell pepper, mushrooms, potatoes, tomatoes, zucchini	beans, chicken, fish, pork	marinades, salad dressings, sauces, soups, stews	basil, bay leaves, chili powder, cilantro, cumin, dill weed, garlic powder, parsley, rosemary, tarragon, thyme
Paprika	sweet, warm	bell pepper, broccoli, cauliflower, potatoes, squash	chicken, shrimp, tofu	marinades, rice, salad dressings, sauces, soups, stews	cayenne pepper, chili powder, cinnamon, cumin, dill weed, garlic powder
Dill weed	earthy, sweet	cabbage, carrots, cucumbers, green beans, potatoes, tomatoes	cheese, chicken, eggs, fish	breads, egg dishes, salad dressings, sandwiches, sauces, soups, tuna salad	basil, coriander, cumin, garlic, mint, mustard seeds, oregano, paprika, parsley, tarragon

Continued on page 72

Herbs and Spices: Your Way

Continued from page 71

Italian seasoning	earthy	asparagus, bell pepper, mushrooms, squash, tomatoes, zucchini	chicken, ground beef, fish, white beans	dips, fish, marinades, meatballs, pasta sauce, salad dressings, soups, stews	lemon
Celery seed	slightly bitter, celery-like flavor	cabbage, cauliflower, cucumber, pickled vegetables, potatoes, tomatoes	cheese, chicken dishes, fish, meatloaf	breads, coleslaw dressing, egg salad, potato salad, salad dressings	cilantro, cumin, garlic, ginger, mustard seeds, parsley, rosemary, thyme
Parsley	earthy	carrots, eggplant, mushrooms, parsnips, potatoes, turnips, zucchini	beef, chicken, fish, tofu	salad dressings, sauces, marinades	basil, bay leaves, celery seed, dill weed, garlic powder, oregano, rosemary, tarragon, thyme
Mint	sweet	carrots, cucumber, eggplant, mushrooms, potatoes, tomatoes, zucchini	beans, lentils	marinades, yogurt sauces, cucumber salad	cilantro, dill weed
Cilantro	sweet, warm	avocado, tomatoes, onion, bell pepper, citrus fruits, corn	chicken, fish, lentils, shrimp, tofu	burgers, guacamole, marinades, salads, salsas, soups, topping for tacos	celery seed, coriander, cumin, garlic powder, mint, oregano
All-purpose seasoning	spicy	asparagus, parsnips, squash, zucchini	chicken, beef, pork, seafood	burgers, chicken, deviled eggs, fish, pork, salad dressings, soups	lemon
Chili powder	spicy	corn, green beans, potatoes, squash, tomatoes	beans, beef, chicken, fish	marinades, salad dressings, sauces, soups	basil, oregano, paprika
Tarragon	spicy	artichokes, carrots, mushrooms, potatoes, spinach	beef, cheese, chicken, eggs, fish	marinades, mayonnaise, salad dressings	basil, bay leaves, dill weed, garlic powder, oregano, parsley, thyme

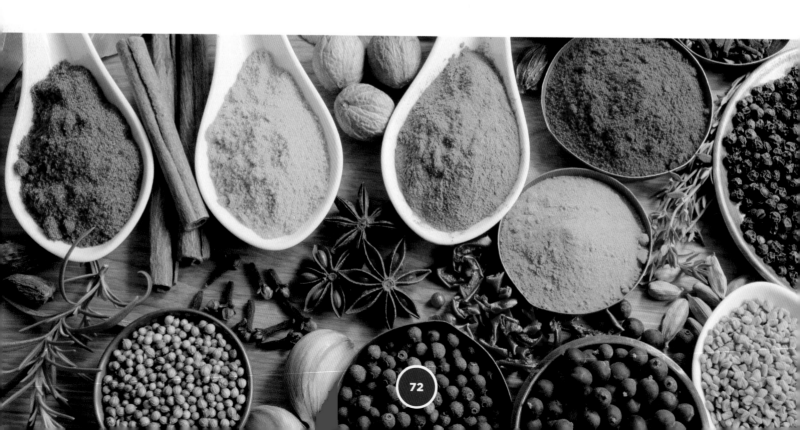

Basic Home Cooking Skills

Roasting a Chicken

INGREDIENTS:

1   whole chicken
1   tablespoon butter
2   cloves of garlic, smashed
1   lemon, cut in half
    Salt and pepper to your liking

Roasting a whole chicken is easy and cheaper than buying breasts, thighs and other pieces. By using a whole chicken, you can make several meals and also make chicken stock for another meal or two. Follow this basic recipe to start, then try adding herbs and spices to the butter to make it your own recipe.

DIRECTIONS:
Preheat oven to 400 degrees F.

Remove the giblets and neck from the chicken. Often, these parts are packaged and left in the neck or body cavity. Rub the entire chicken with butter. Sprinkle with salt and pepper.

Stuff the garlic and lemon halves into the chicken's body cavity. Tie the drumsticks (legs) together with a piece of clean kitchen string.

Place the chicken in a roasting pan or an oven-proof skillet and cook in the oven for 1 hour. Use a meat thermometer to make sure the chicken is at 165 degrees F.

Let the chicken rest for at least 10 minutes. Remove lemon and string; discard. Carve and serve.

Use the chopped giblets and neck to add flavor to stock, soups or gravy. Cook the parts covered in stock or cold water. Bring to a boil, then reduce heat to medium low and simmer for about one hour. Once cooked fully, the parts should be easy to chop. Again, make sure the chicken parts are cooked to at least 165 degrees F.

WARNING: Because of possible harmful bacteria in raw chicken, be sure to thoroughly wash hands, all utensils and any surfaces the chicken may have touched.

Making Chicken Stock: Your Way
After you have eaten all the meat, you can make chicken stock from the leftover carcass.

To make chicken stock:
In a large pot with a lid, cover chicken carcass with cold water. Bring to a boil, then reduce heat to medium low and simmer for at least 4 hours. You can also add herbs, vegetable ends or peels to the stock while it cooks. Strain the stock and discard solids (including the solid fat on the surface). Store in a lidded container in the refrigerator for 2-3 days or in the freezer for up to 3 months.

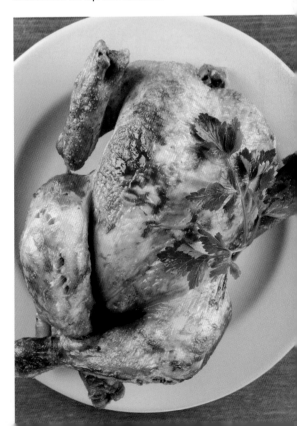

Basic Home Cooking Skills

8 Basic Ways to Prepare Eggs

1. **Hard-boiled.** Yolk is completely set and pale yellow. Cover eggs in a pan with cold water, bring to a boil, cover with lid and let sit off heat for 8-12 minutes. Run eggs under cold water to stop cooking then roll them on counter to crack shells. Peel them under running water.

2. **Soft-boiled.** Yolk is runny and slightly unset. Cover eggs in a pan with cold water, bring to a boil, cover with a lid and let sit off heat for 2-3 minutes. To eat, crack off the end of the shell, and scoop out the inside of the egg with a spoon.

3. **Poached.** Runny but warm and thickened yolk and fully set white. Add a splash of vinegar to a pan of simmering water, crack an egg and gently slide it into water without breaking the yolk. Cook until white sets, then scoop out with a slotted spoon and drain on a paper towel.

4. **Sunny-side up.** Top of egg is barely set with an unbroken yolk. Crack into melted butter over medium heat, and cover the pan when you can no longer see through the whites. Cook 4 more minutes.

5. **Fried eggs**, including over-hard (fully cooked yolk), over-medium (almost solid but still runny yolk); and over-easy (runny yolk). Crack into melted butter over medium heat, flip after you can no longer see through the whites, and cook 3 minutes (over-hard), 2 minutes (over-medium), and 1 minute (over-easy).

6. **Scrambled.** Crack an egg, add salt, whisk egg, then cook in melted butter in nonstick skillet, stirring slowly to make large, fluffy curds.

7. **Omelet.** Use a fork or whisk to beat eggs until yolks and whites are mixed. Cook in melted butter in small nonstick skillet over medium heat. Add filling of choice when eggs are firm on the bottom but still runny on top. Cook until eggs are heated through. Fold the omelet in half and roll or slide onto a plate.

8. **Eggs in a basket or eggs in a hole.** Eggs are fried in a hole made in a slice of bread.

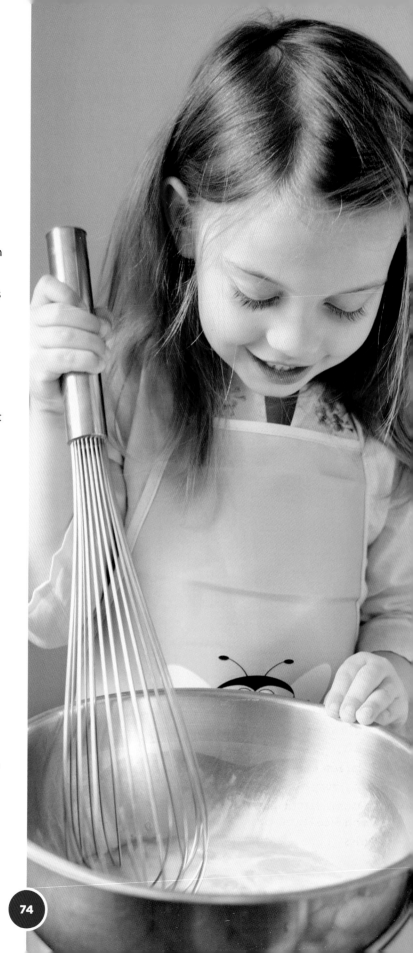

RECIPE INDEX